FOOTBALL

AND

BOOBS

His Playbook For
Her Breast Implants

Dallas Davis

With Vip Dev, M.D.

Football and Boobs

His Playbook For Her Breast Implants

ISBN 978-0-9830536-9-9

Author: Dallas Davis

Book design by WordPros at Elance.com

Front cover: The lady who inspired this book, Jane, in Hawaii

Special thanks go out to Jane, Joy, Jean, Jigger, Jeff, Jim, JL, Lisa, Guy, Vip, Anne, Samantha, Diedre, Nicole, Steve, Barber, Nelson, and all my other wonderful friends who encouraged and inspired me. I couldn't have done this without you.

To The Reader

Hey There–

How is it going? I hope all is well.

If you're reading this book, then your woman is thinking about getting breast implants. That's exciting!

If you two decide that you're happy with what she already has, great! There's nothing better than agreeing that she really is perfect how she is. She'll feel better and so will you. Your relationship will improve because of this.

On the other hand, if she decides to go through with the boob job, you are in for an adventure! Breast implants will not only give you more to look at and play with, but they will give your woman a new source of confidence that will pay off in ways you'd never believe! This too has great potential to improve the health of your relationship.

As men, we are used to being "in charge" and always knowing what to do. We take pride in being able to handle any situation. Change is a bit scary, and breast implants are a change that few men know how to handle.

That's why I'm here. My lady got breast implants a short while ago, and I want you to learn from my experience.

Since I'm not a surgeon, I'm not going to use a bunch of medical mumbo jumbo. To make it easier to understand, I've translated everything you need to know into terms you can understand: FOOTBALL. That's right, I'll teach you all you need to know in pigskin words.

If you know what a quarterback is and have ever seen a long bomb throw right before the buzzer, you can understand this book!

On the other hand, I want to make sure that you can trust the information I provide. That's why I've joined forces with noted plastic surgeon Dr. Vip Dev. In bite-sized chunks, this former football-playing surgeon shares the perspective he's gained from performing hundreds of breast augmentations.

Keep reading and you will learn the ins and outs of boob jobs. You'll find out the secrets that will help YOU help HER get the best breasts possible!

More importantly, you'll understand your woman better and learn how to help her become the hottest woman she can be.

That's right.....

       Cleavage...

           Big full cups...

And a confident girl who will FEEL sexier and BE sexier with YOU!

How can your relationship NOT get better?!?

Remember, breast implants are a big time, money, and pain investment. The information in this book will help you to help your woman get great breasts. You just have to read it and apply it. Then enjoy your life with your bustier woman!

Breast Wishes,

Dallas

Dallas Davis

Dallas@FootballAndBoobs.com
facebook.com/FootballAndBoobs
twitter.com/FootballNBoobs

Disclaimer

This book is intended to provide helpful and informative material on the subject of breast augmentation in an entertaining style. It is sold with the understanding that the author, publisher, and any contributors are not engaged in providing medical, health, psychological, or any other kind of personal professional services in the book. It merely intends to help potential breast augmentation patients and their significant others understand some of the potential effects of surgery, the types of decisions to be made, and what factors may be involved. Any decisions are to be made by the patient only.

Do not use any information in this book to diagnose or treat any condition or complication. Again, this book is not offering medical advice. For any and all issues or questions, always contact a trained medical professional.

This book is not meant to substitute for communication with competent medical professionals. Instead, it is meant to help enable understanding and foster better communication.

While it is the author's hope that this book can assist in communication between men and women, neither he nor the publisher take responsibility for any reader employing the techniques, conversational strategies, or exact phrasing contained herein. The reader is assumed to be an adult who can decide what to say or do.

In no way does this book imply that plastic surgery can heal any cracks in a relationship. In fact, it can have the opposite effect. If there are serious relationship issues, please contact a trained counselor.

The author, publisher, and contributors specifically disclaim all responsibility for any liability, loss, or risk, personal or otherwise, that is incurred as a consequence, directly or indirectly, of the use and application of the contents of this book.

References herein to any NFL teams or players are for illustrative purposes only; no endorsement of *Football and Boobs* by the NFL, NFL teams, or NFL players, or of specific information or techniques it describes, is suggested or intended. This book is independently authored and published and is not sponsored, endorsed by, or otherwise affiliated with the NFL or other aforementioned entities.

Unless a photograph is explicitly marked as being "Patient ##", it is a photograph of a model only, not a patient of Dr. Vip Dev.

OK, now that that's out of the way, let's get to the good stuff.

Table of Contents

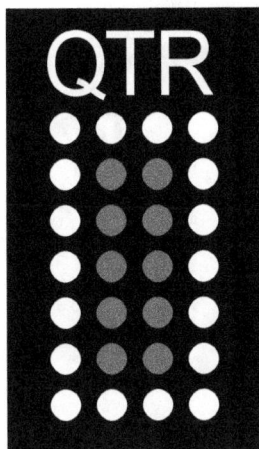

QTR

Pre-Game:

Intro

Questions This Section Answers:

What is this book all about?

Why did this Dallas guy write this book?

* 1 *

What Is This Book All About?

This book is for you, sir. This book is all about you and your relationship with the woman in your life. She's your lady, and has been for some time. Over those days, weeks, months, or years, your relationship has transformed. It's continually changed, subtly at times, and more significantly at others.

Do you remember that first kiss? Or the first time you saw her take off her shirt? These are relationship accelerators, causing change.

Now, your woman has presented you with the fact that she's thinking about changing herself, which will inevitably affect your relationship.

If you're like most men, your knowledge of breast implants is limited to what you've seen in Playboy, late night Cinemax movies, or the internet. This probably has tainted your view of breast implants one way or the other. **You have many misconceptions. You need more information.**

Breast augmentation can affect many aspects of your relationship: emotions, physical looks and feel, family, and finances.

You will discover how **breast implants could affect your woman's emotions, self-esteem, and health.** You'll discover how it may affect YOUR emotions too.

It's not just the stark difference in her appearance before and after surgery that will change things in her mind and yours. The entire process

This book's aim is to give you a clear understanding of what breast implants may mean to your woman, to you, and to your relationship.

of breast augmentation and recovery will be an emotional ride that will hopefully *draw the two of you closer together*. However, if you say the wrong things, it could drive you further apart.

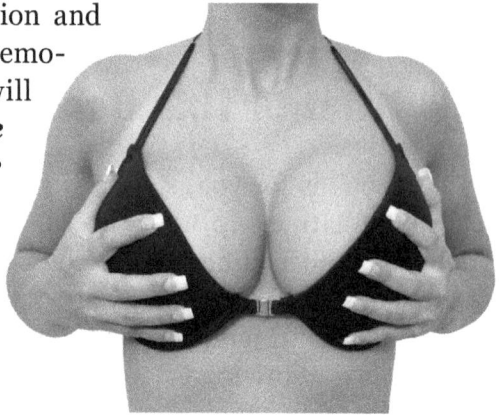

You'll discover *how breast implants could affect her physically* (for better or worse), and how this physical change can lead to a more—ahem—physical relationship between you two.

Depending on your relationship, you may have a family, with or without children. The *health risks* involved in breast augmentation (like any surgery) can have significant effects on your family. You'll learn which of these risks are real and just how many are just myths.

Breast augmentation is by no means an inexpensive process. Someone will be paying a considerable amount of money for the surgery and for all the various other expenses. You'll learn about the *costs of breast augmentation*, both expected and unexpected. These expenses include TIME, of which you will be spending a lot.

Can you see now why breast implants can cause a huge change (for good or bad) in your relationship?

Don't worry. By the time you reach the end of this book, you'll know all you need to help her get the best breasts for her, you, and your relationship.

Even though *this book is meant for men*, it is also *aimed to help women understand men's thought process* before, during, and after surgery.

This book also *enables women to communicate with*

4

their men better about the topic of breast augmentation. Put it in his hands and ask him to read it... he will. If you are a woman who has purchased this book, but know your man never reads, you can use the football metaphor to explain breast augmentation to him.

Ladies, please remember the language is geared toward guys. Please do not take offense to any of the "locker room language".

Now guys, are you ready? I'll start with what I know best...

How Does Dallas Know?

My name is Dallas Davis, and I am a "boob man". ("Hi, Dallas" is your response.)

I never really thought I was a "boob man" to be honest. I always prided myself on liking a girl's intelligence, her pretty face, her smooth legs, or even her round butt.

Having always been athletic, I like fit women. Fit women typically don't have large breasts.

There are some out there—God bless 'em—that have big breasts to go with their long legs, round butts, and tight abs. But those are few and far between.

I've dated many women. All had pretty faces, most were intelligent, and lots of them sported great legs. Some of them had asses so nice they'd make J-Lo turn green with envy.

But I never dated a girl with big breasts. Sure there was a date or two and some random hookups, but never did I ever get exclusive with the owner of a set of giant breasts.

Don't get me wrong. I won't lie. I am a man. A nice set of breasts always got my attention, wherever I was. I couldn't hide from it.

By now, I've seen more than my fair share of them up close. I've played with enough breasts to get the "3-second thumb-forefinger bra-clasp opening" method down pat.

I know some guys who are so boob-centric that they won't date a girl smaller than a B-cup. They just aren't attracted to them. That's a loss for them, because there are so many great women out there with smaller chests.

When I started dating Jane, I was fine with her boobs. They weren't tiny, but they weren't anything worth telling my buddies about either.

She was so cool and so fun and smart, that I didn't really care that she barely filled up my not-so-large hands. They were cute and perky boobs. The fact that she didn't have larger breasts didn't matter to me.

She had plenty of sexy to go around. She was in great shape, had sexy tattoos, and looked great in a bikini.

We had many months of happy times in and out of the bedroom. Having kissed and caressed them often, never once did I think to complain about her boobs.

Sitting on her bed one night after dinner, came "The Talk"...

"I'm thinking about getting a boob job. What do you think?"

To be honest, I was caught off guard by this. I thought, "Seriously?! A boob job? Why? I like your breasts!".

Then she explained it to me.

She wasn't getting the implants for me.

She wasn't getting them so that she could get another man.

She wanted them to make HERSELF happy. She wanted to feel more like a woman. She too had been brainwashed by years of the media's insistence that "boobs = woman". (Although she didn't say it in so many words!)

I told her she was beautiful, sexy, and womanly. She didn't care what I thought. It was all about what was *inside her head.*

She knew she could spend thousands of dollars and years of her life on some therapist's couch talking about why she didn't feel sexy. Or she could just spend some of her hard-earned cash and make her body look much sexier in her eyes. She earned it, she saved it, and she had the right to spend her money how she wanted.

I asked her about the surgery, and she knew all the details. I asked her about the costs and risks, and she showed me a stack of printouts from the internet. She then showed me her legal pad full of her own research and detailed notes.

She had done her homework. She knew what she was getting into. I had to respect that.

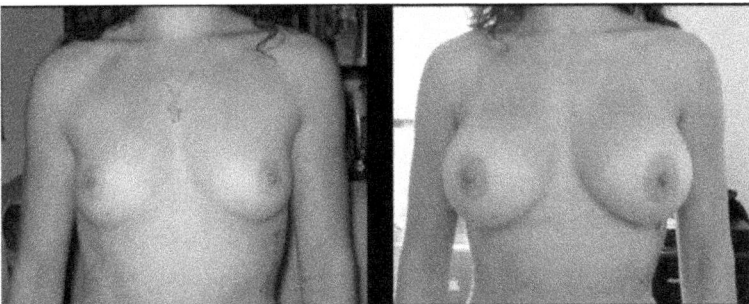

She had done her homework. She knew what she was getting into. I had to respect that.

What could I say? Never in a million years would I have thought I'd be dating a woman with breast implants. But I am an open-minded guy. It was her body, her money, and ultimately, her decision.

She decided to go forward with the surgery. That was a big decision. While I could have bailed, I chose to stick with her and support her through the whole process. Because I did this, I was able to learn a lot about the breast implant decision-making process.

Before   **After (1 year)**

7

I helped her work out some of the details before the surgery, and I took care of her after the surgery. It wasn't always fun and it wasn't always pretty, but I learned the best ways to deal with her painful, emotional, long recovery.

I am so glad that she chose to get breast augmentation. Not only does she looks better with her shirt off, but she looks a lot better in her clothes too. That's because first, most modern fashions are designed to look good on women with reasonably large boobs and second (and more importantly), she has a ton more confidence.

That confidence transformed our sex life and took it to a new level.

If you can't tell, I was thrilled! She was happy with the results, and I was too. We talked more, our sex life got better, and it helped our relationship.

You too can have this. You just need a little help from someone who's been there before.

You will quickly grasp what I took months to learn, both from my experience and my research. You will also benefit from the experiences of other men sharing their knowledge with you.

Keep reading, and you will learn everything a man needs know about breast implants from the all-to-familiar framework of football.

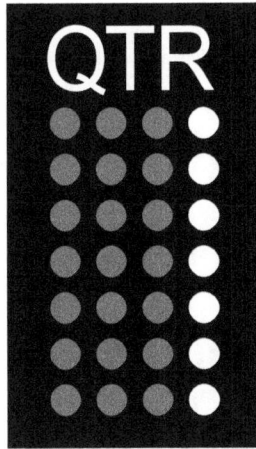

FIRST QUARTER:

GETTING THE INFO

Questions this Section Answers:

What does **football** have to do with breast implants?

Just **what is a boob job** anyway?

What will her augmented boobs **look** like?

What will her new breasts **feel** like?

Should I care **WHY she want implants**?

What are the **health risks** of a boob job?

How much will breast augmentation **cost**?

What is the **time investment** of a boob job?

* 2 *

Breasts and The Game of Your Life

Many American men believe that life happens four quarters at a time, on a grass rectangle. While it can be very easy to be obsessed with football, the truth is that there is a bigger game that matters more – *Your Life!*

That's right, your life is the most important thing you have. How you spend each day matters more than the outcome of any playoff or rivalry game there is. This might be hard for some to swallow (especially for Alabama and Auburn fans), but it's true.

A large part of your life is how you and your woman interact. The health of that relationship can significantly impact your well-being.

Think about it. If your career is going great and your team is on a 7-game winning streak, life still won't feel right if there is friction between you and your woman.

One of the only ways to win at the game of life is to have a great teammate and partner to help you along. You need a winning relationship to have a winning life.

If you are anything like me, when you play a game, you play to WIN!

Winning in the relationship stage of the game of life requires that you have a happy, healthy woman who loves you. If she is unhappy with herself, she can never be the happy, healthy, loving woman you need.

So, your woman has told you about her desire for breast implants. This presents a new situation in your game of life and sets the stage for this book...

The Game Situation You Face

Your team of two (you and your woman) battled against the world through nearly two quarters. You just got the ball back.

It's first and ten, and you're on your own ten-yard line. There are four seconds left before half-time.

Your team has a choice to make.

You can take the safe route, and kneel the ball. Your team will go into half-time, and come up with a better game plan for the rest of the game. This decision is perfect if you're happy with where you are and don't want to risk losing what you have.

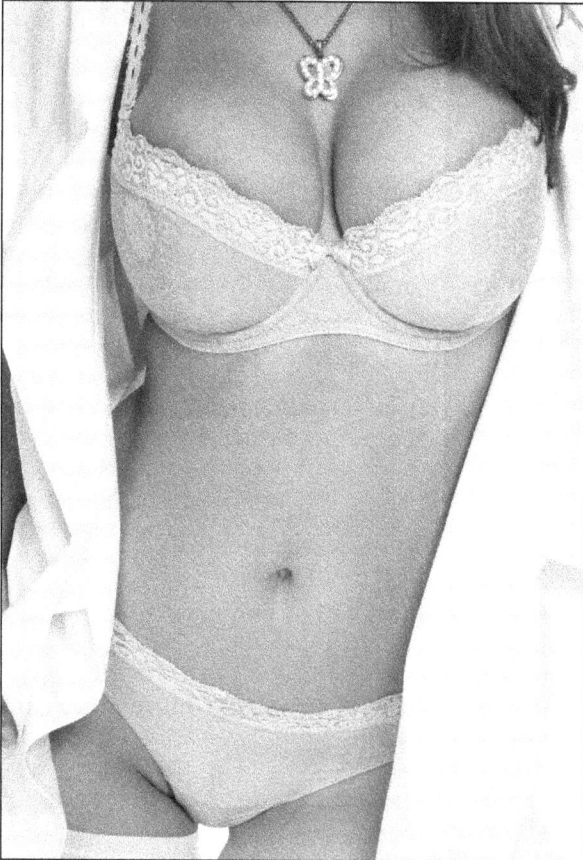

Or...

You can take advantage of your opportunity and try to score a big touchdown! By going for the touchdown, your team will be taking a risk, but you could also be setting yourselves up to get a lot closer to winning the game.

Think about how scoring a big touchdown right before the half expires could give your team momentum going into the second half of the game!

Right now, your two-person team in the game of life has just called a timeout to talk it over.

You will both have to come to a decision soon about whether or not to go for the deep pass play and how exactly your team will execute this play.

(In other words, your woman will decide whether or not she will get breast implants, and will work with a surgeon to decide the various details involved in breast augmentation.)

This is the game of life you are playing. The goal is to have a happy relationship with a woman who enjoys her body, whether her breasts are natural or enhanced.

Breast augmentation MAY be able to help you win in the game of life or it may not.

The rest of this book is based on making the decision to go for it (breast augmentation) or not, and if you choose to go for it, how the play (surgery) will go down.

* **3** *

Who Are the Players?

You can think of the breast augmentation surgery and recovery process as one big "pass play". There's a quarterback, a center, a wide receiver, a play call, the ball, the opponents, and the coaches. You need to know each one's role.

In this pass play, the quarterback will decide either to go for it or not, and will then choose the play. Then, the quarterback will snap the ball and throw a pass to the wide receiver. Meanwhile, the center is blocking to protect the quarterback from the opponents. And there is a coach on the sidelines helping you along the whole way.

Doesn't this all sound a little familiar?

The Quarterback: Your Woman

In the game of boobs, there is no person more important than your woman. She is the quarterback.

She will have the final say on whether or not she wants to have the surgery. Your woman will decide which surgeon she will let operate on her. She will work with the surgeon to decide on what she wants her new breasts to look like.

She is the ultimate decision maker.

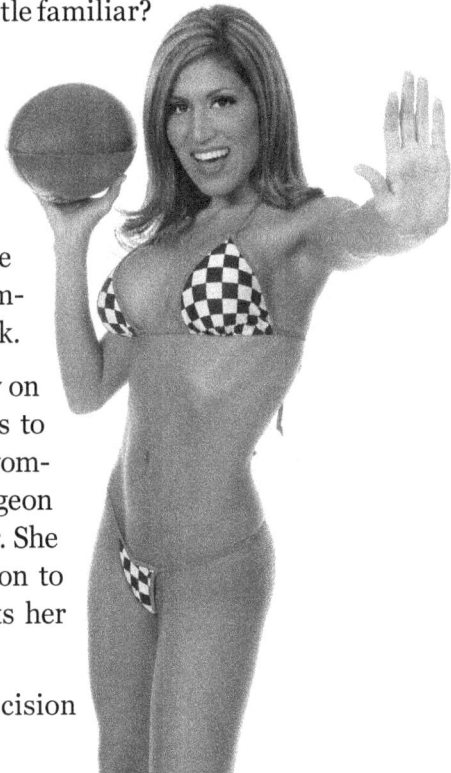

Wide Receiver: The Plastic Surgeon

Since the 1960s, the forward pass has been the dominant mode of high-scoring offenses in both college and pro football. Having good wide receivers is essential to having a good passing game.

In the boob game, the plastic surgeon is the wide receiver. It's "in his hands".

He or she (most commonly male, so we will stick with "he") will be operating on your woman's chest. His skill and technique control about 50% of how this "pass play" goes.

Once your woman—the QB—has selected the right surgeon and goes in for the surgery, it's up to him to make your woman's breasts the best, given the material he has to start with.

The Center: You

No pass play works unless the quarterback has time to throw the pass. The offensive line has to provide protection.

In this case, that's you. Your job is to keep your woman safe. You are the center.

Your job is to help protect her from all the opponents that are trying to bring her down, while at the same time staying out of her way. It's a tricky thing to do, but it will be worth it for you.

Also, she may also ask for your suggestions. Think of it like Peyton Manning asking Jeff Saturday whether or not they should go for it, and what play to run. Jeff can only suggest. He can't make the decision.

QBs greatly appreciate their linemen. You'll be the one who benefits the most from her beautiful new assets! You'll enjoy your new toys if you do your job right!

The Opponents: Complications and Negative Energy

There are plenty of forces that can keep you from scoring the touchdown. The opposing team is made up of "complications" and "negative energy".

There are a ton of different types of surgical complications. Some can happen during or right after the surgery, and some can develop over time.

Later in the book, you will learn more about the complications that might pop up, how to recognize them, and what to do to fight them off.

There are other players on the defense that will try to stop you from winning the game. These opponents are known as "negative energy", and can take many forms.

These can be family members or even random people who will try to convince your woman not to have surgery. They will try telling her horror stories or may tell her she is doing something morally wrong by getting breast implants.

Let her get all the facts, and make a well-informed decision. But don't let ignorant people who have done no research influence her by attacking her emotions.

...don't let ignorant people who have done no research influence her by attacking her emotions.

Negative energy can also take the form of fear. Any time you, or more importantly, your woman gets afraid or nervous about the surgery, you need to help bring both of your spirits back up. That's your job! Look back at the facts of the surgery and check out the great results other women have experienced.

One of the first things people notice about Dr. Vip Dev is that he's
a big guy with a big heart, an easy
smile, and a warmth and genuine
spirit that puts everybody at ease.

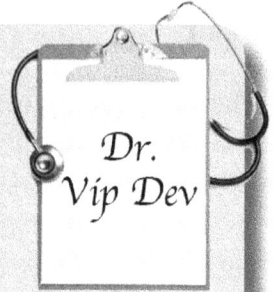

*Dr.
Vip Dev*

A former football player, he became a plastic surgeon out of a deep desire to make positive changes
in people's lives. Providing both aesthetic and reconstructive care gives
him the opportunity to
impact patients of vir-
tually every age and
station in life.

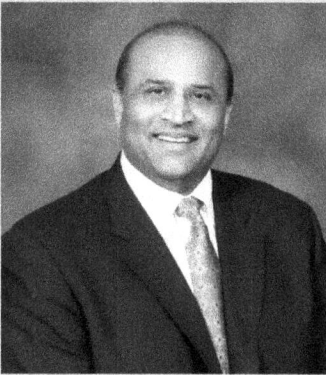

Dr. Vip Dev trained in
plastic & reconstruc-
tive surgery at the
University of Texas at
San Antonio Health
Sciences Center after
completing his MD degree at Ross University and
studying Medical Ethics at Oxford and Biomedical
Sciences at the University of Pennsylvania.

While his patients call him "Dr. Dev", in this book
I refer to him as "Dr. Vip" because (1) he's a per-
sonable, first-name kind of guy and (2) he really
was a Very Important Person (VIP) at making this
book happen.

You can learn more at his website *www.vipmd.com*.

*(Examples of Dr. Vip Dev's surgical procedures
can be seen in the Appendix.)*

The Coach: Me

No team plays without someone who's been there before and understands the game better than they do. They always have a coach.

I am here to help you as you help your woman get those glorious boobs. I am your coach. Read the rest of this book, and use it as your playbook.

I am also available for free 15-minute private consultations. Send me an email at:

Dallas@FootballAndBoobs.com

and we can arrange a call. In this coaching session, you can tell me about your situation in as much detail as you are comfortable with. I can either just lend an ear to let you vent your frustrations and fears, or I can work with you about a game plan for where to go from there.

My advice to you is only advice from the perspective of a man who's been there before.

Remember that a surgeon is the best person to give your woman advice on what choices she should make for her surgery and her recovery.

What are the Playing Conditions?

In week 12 of the 2007 NFL season, the Dolphins visited the Steelers in some of the worst playing conditions in recent history.

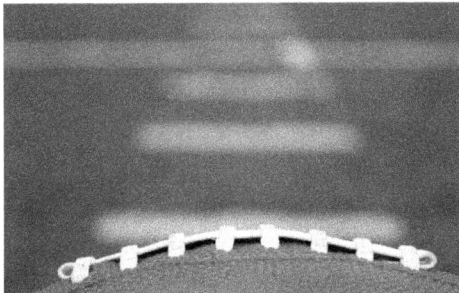

The Pittsburgh sky dumped so much rain on the field that the game was delayed 25 minutes and the yard-lines had to be repainted right before the game. Players were slipping on the mud and sinking into puddles so much that the offenses just couldn't get going. At one point, Miami punted from their own end zone, and when the ball hit the ground, it DIDN'T BOUNCE! The punt stuck in the mud!

Pittsburgh scored the only points of the game by field goal with 17 seconds left in the game, and went home with a 3-0 victory. In this case, the playing conditions dictated what the players could do throughout each play of the game.

The field on which your boobie play will go down is your woman's body. Her natural anatomy will dictate what can or cannot be done surgically.

Your woman's exact body size and shape will impact what she can expect after the surgery. The plastic surgeon will work with her on her expectations and suggest what he thinks is best.

What is the Play Call?

To successfully work as a team, an offense must know where everyone is going. This keeps the players focused and prevents them from running into one another.

In this "implant pass play", all the players need to be on the same page. You all need to agree on who's doing what, and how exactly the play will be run.

There are many specific play call decisions to make, and these

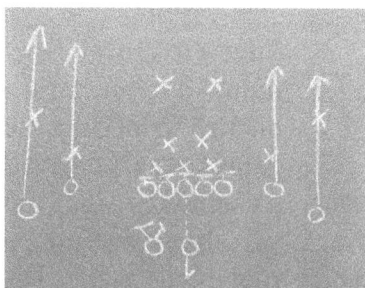

are outlined in the "Second Quarter" of this book.

These decisions include picking the implant type, the incision location, the implant shape, where the implant sits in her body, and the approximate size of the implant.

* **4** *

What is a Boob Job?

There are many types of breast surgery. Breasts can be made bigger, made smaller, lifted, or removed.

Types of Breast Surgery

Obviously this book is mostly about making breast bigger, also known as "breast augmentation" or in medical-mumbo-jumbo, "augmentation mammoplasty".

Breast reduction surgery (aka "reduction mammoplasty") helps some women improve their quality of life by reducing the amount of breast tissue they have. Women who get this procedure typically have experienced back pain, social stigmatization, and/or limited physical activities due to their large breasts.

Some women have the misfortune of developing breast cancer. To treat this horrible disease, doctors may recommend they undergo surgery to remove breast tissue, such as lumpectomy (cancerous tissue only removal), quadrantectomy (partial breast removal) or mastectomy (whole breast removal). Women who undergo single- or double- mastectomies will often elect to have breast augmentation after the initial surgery has healed. Post-mastectomy augmentation is more involved and may require multiple procedures. On the other hand, it is becoming more and more common for surgeons to perform breast reconstruction immediately after removal.

Another surgery sometimes done in conjunction with breast augmentation

Another surgery sometimes done in conjunction with breast augmentation is a breast lift.

is a breast lift. Also known as "mastoplexy", a breast lift involves removing part of the breast tissue and skin to help re-position the nipple and make the breast look less droopy or saggy.

Now back to the type of "boob job" that you are most interested in...

The Basic Breast Augmentation Process

Technically known as a "breast augmentation" or "BA", a boob job is a surgical procedure that involves inserting prosthetic implants into a woman's chest.

It sounds simple, but in actuality it's much more complicated than that. You should know the basics of a boob job procedure.

Before the surgery, your woman will be sedated and given anesthesia so that she doesn't feel the pain of the operation. She will either be totally unconscious from "general anesthesia" or put in a strange semi-conscious state called "twilight sedation", in which she won't feel pain or remember the operation but can respond to the doctor. Once you read the rest of this section, you'll understand why.

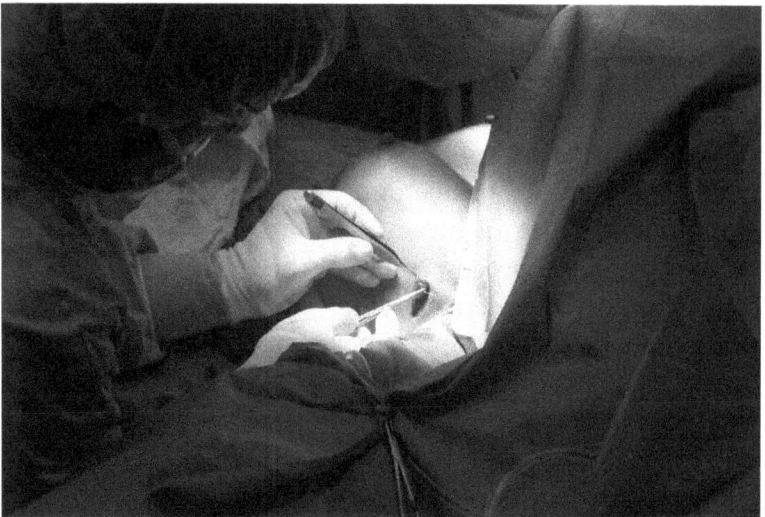

Believe it or not, your lady's breasts do not naturally have an "implant insertion hole" in them. And guess what!? They don't have a big empty spot on the inside of them just waiting to be filled with an implant. These holes have to be made, which is where the surgery part kicks in.

While surgical techniques vary from surgeon to surgeon and continually improve as technology progresses, the basics are the same.

First, the doctor uses a scalpel to make the insertion hole, whether it's on the breast itself or in some other place. (Yes, the hole can be in another spot... more on that later.) While it's uncommon, if the surgeon messes up the incision, it can leave a bad scar.

He then has to use some tools to make "the pocket" into which the implant will be placed. This step is rather serious, as it involves separating the breast tissue from the muscle, or the muscle from other muscle, or connective tissue from muscle.

This part involves skill on the surgeon's part. If he doesn't make the pockets the right size and shape, the new boobs may end up hanging unevenly or pointing in different directions.

The surgeon then inserts the implants, adjusts them, and moves things around as he sees fit. Once he gets them how he wants them, he sews up the incisions and applies bandages.

Finally, the surgeon or a nurse may wrap up the boobs, chest, and upper back with a bunch of tight wrapping. It looks a lot like the ace bandage you use to wrap your sore knee after that Thanksgiving day family pigskin game. Then again, the surgeon may declare her ready to go home wearing nothing more than a t-shirt or surgical bra.

The patient will rest for a while in the "recovery room" under supervision before you or her caretaker will be allowed to take her home.

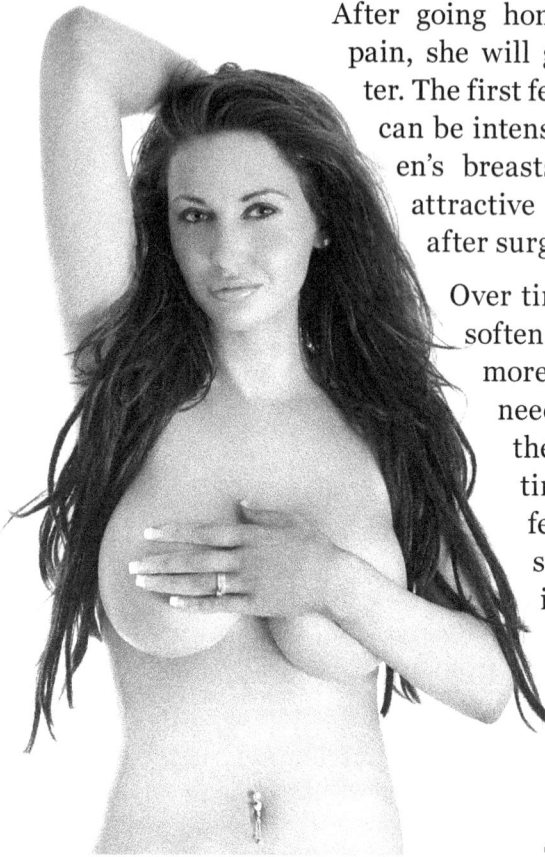

After going home groggy and in pain, she will gradually feel better. The first few days of recovery can be intense, and most women's breasts don't look very attractive for days or weeks after surgery.

Over time, her boobs will soften and begin to look more natural. She will need to go back to see the surgeon a few times over the next few months to make sure things are going well.

It will probably take months for her breasts to finally settle into their final state.

Those are the basics of a standard boob job. Of course, the details of various techniques fill thousands pages of medical journals. Aren't you glad you don't have to read all that? Just read the rest of this book!

* 5 *

What Do Augmented Breasts Look Like?

I bet you want to know about what your woman's breast might look like if you two decide to "go for it".

A lot of men have negative misconceptions about what breasts with implants in them look like. Once you acknowledge that you *think you know* what augmented breasts look like, you can then open your mind to be surprised by just how good they can look. Let's get the negative breast implant images out of your head.

The Implants You've Seen

Most guys see breast implants in one of two places, strip clubs and porn.

If you're like almost every man I know, you've seen your fair share of porn. And I bet you've come across plenty of videos or photos of women with terribly fake-looking boob jobs.

You know what I mean. Sometimes, it looks like someone cut a grapefruit in half, bolted both halves to a woman's chest, and then drew on nipples.

Other girls will have fake knockers that are so unbelievably big that you wonder where they keep the wheelbarrow to haul them around in.

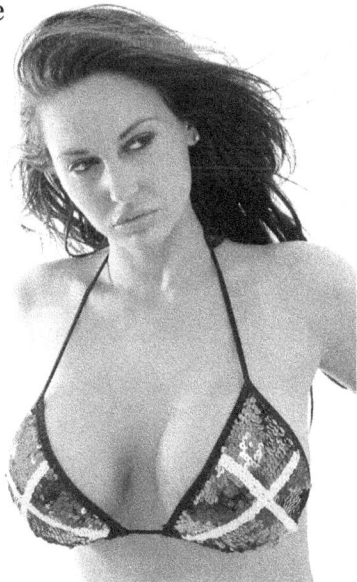

25

Some girls' boobs are so far apart, you swear they need a titanium bra three sizes too small to give them any cleavage.

The worst are the girls who have big scars on their boobs and are dumb enough to let the photographers take pictures from angles that prominently feature those scars or who dance on stage and hang them over your face. Yuck!

It makes sense that out of all of the sets of augmented breasts you've seen, a lot are ugly porn/stripper boobs.

But is porn really a reliable indicator of what your woman's new breasts might look like?

Think about it. If a woman is in a situation where stripping or doing porn is a good financial move, she probably can't afford to get a high-quality breast augmentation from a good surgeon. She likely had to go to a bargain basement surgeon. Also, since breast implants can be costly, many of these girls have to get "back to work" too soon after the surgery (before fully healing).

That's the bad news.

The good news is that you've probably also seen a lot of fake breasts that you thought were real because the look just like phenomenal natural breasts. You just didn't realize it. That's right, some boob jobs are so good that they look real!

The Breasts You Both Want

As you've probably found out in the bedroom, not all women are porn stars. They don't all have sex like porn stars and they don't all look like porn stars.

Some women who seek breast implants **want** to look like porn stars. They desire this hyper-sexualized image and want very large, very round breasts

However, many ladies wanting breast augmentation don't want to look like this; they want to achieve a look that is more natural. Some women just want to get average-sized "no-one-would-ever-suspect-implants" breasts, while others want "larger-than-average-yet-natural-looking" breasts.

Your woman will need to decide what "look" she wants. A good surgeon can give your woman a glaringly obvious, attention-grabbing set of breasts; a very subtle, totally natural augmentation; or breasts somewhere in between that look large but natural.

That's right, she can get boobs that look so amazing that even women who see her changing in the gym locker room will swear they are real!

You and your woman should discuss what she's looking for. Since your goal is a happy woman and a happy relationship, her desires are most important. But since you will have to live with her decision, you can express your opinion (as long as you don't mind if she ignores it).

Work with her and support her decision about the image she wants so that she can get the breasts you both want. No matter what, she will get more luscious boobs, and you will get to look at and play with them!

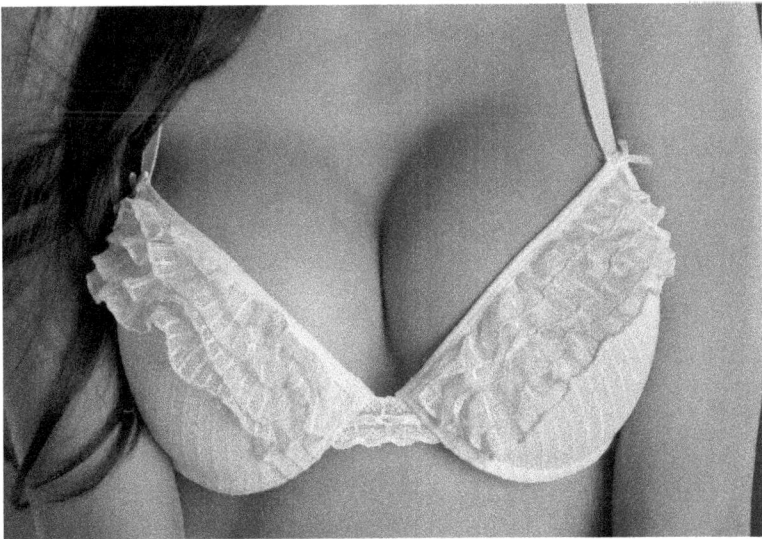

Bigger... Duh? But What Else?

Obviously, after getting implants, her breasts will look noticeably bigger. This will especially be true in the first month or two post-op, when they will be very swollen from the trauma of the surgery.

Just like blowing up that clown face balloon for your nephew makes his nose stretch out all funny, increasing your woman's breast size with implants will stretch out her skin and each areolae (the dark areas around her nipples). Don't be surprised if she goes from having small ones to big ones. Then again, some women's areolae don't change at all.

Also, because the skin is stretched by the implant, the veins in her breasts may be more visible after the surgery. Be prepared to see some of the veins in her chest more.

Will There Be Scars on Her Breasts?

The amount of scarring on your woman's breasts depends on a lot of factors, but the number one factor is the method used to insert the implants.

Some insertion methods make zero scars on the breasts, some make small scars, and some make larger scars. The type and size of implant she chooses may force your surgeon to make a bigger or more noticeable incision.

Also, it really matters how skilled the surgeon is. Some are magic, and you would swear a blade never touched the woman. With others, you wonder if they missed the day in kindergarten where they taught you how to cut things.

Additionally, your woman's skin type can make a big difference in the scarring process too. Fair-skinned women tend to have lighter scars, and olive-skinned women tend to have darker scars.

Some women form what are called "keloid scars", which are thick, hard, and dark. If your woman has any nasty scars already, it can give you and her an indication of how her breast augmentation scars might heal.

The bottom line is that there may be some scars or there might not be. Like any other small scar, they will usually fade over time, so don't freak out about scars being there early on. Have patience, my friend! Her new breasts need time but will look great!

Laying Down

When a woman with large natural breasts lays down on her back, her breasts will most likely flatten and move toward her armpits. Since breast implants are self-contained, they don't move in the same way. Because of this, implanted breasts retain their shape more when a woman lies on her back.

Personally, I think it looks sexier this way. There's no "where did they go" that you get with natural breasts in bed.

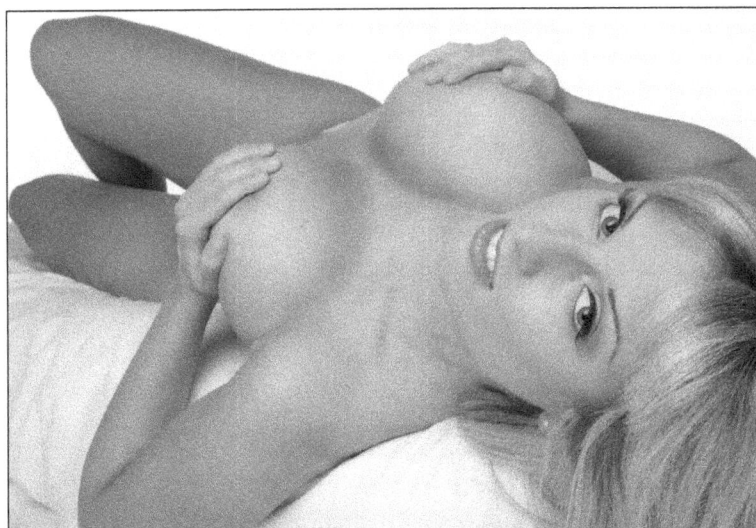

* 6 *

How Will They Feel to the Touch?

Are you thinking, "Looks are one thing. Everybody gets to see her breasts with clothes on. And I am excited to look at them naked. But what I really want to know is how the 'new twins' are going to feel when we are playing in the bedroom?"

If you aren't thinking along those lines, YOU SHOULD BE!

Augmented breasts can feel very much like natural breast tissue... or a lot different.

There's going to be a difference in "feel" depending on which type of implant she chooses. The two kinds of implant filler material are saline and silicone.

Keep reading and you'll learn about all the difference between the implant types.

What matters for now is that saline implant is a bag of salt water, and it will to feel like a bag of water inserted under your girl's existing breast tissue.

If your girl is starting off with about a B-cup or more, then you will feel mostly breast tissue. It shouldn't be a big deal for you. But if she's got less than that to start with, saline implants *may* feel like just a bag of water under skin.

Another factor is the placement of the implant—how many layers of tissue are between it and the skin. More on this later.

Jane got saline implants under her pectoral muscles. She started with a small B-cup and went up to a full D. After a long wait, her breasts started to move and bounce like natural breasts. I could move them around, squish them together, and rub my face in them. Talk about FUN to play with!

As much fun as saline breasts implants can be, silicone implants feel even better. If you just hold one in your hand, you can tell they are squishier, and almost identical to natural breast tissue in texture. Once implanted and fully accepted by a woman's body, they move and bounce and do almost everything like natural boobs.

As much fun as saline breasts implants can be silicone implants feel even better.

Many women choose not to get silicone implants because there are several trade-offs of doing so. Keep reading to find out more.

The bottom line is that unless your girl is starting with "mosquito bites" and gets saline implants, you will likely be happy with the way she fills your hands and how it feels.

Ripples

You might feel or see some "ripples" on the sides and bottoms of her new boobs when she sits in some positions.

The less breast material she has to begin with, the closer to the skin the implants will be. That means that any ripples in the implant will be easily felt through the skin. Saline implants tend to feel "ripply" more often than silicone ones.

If you think that the presence of any ripples on your girl's big new breasts will piss you off, gross you out, or make Mr. Happy go limp, then this could be a big issue later on. Tell her about this now!

Talk to your girl if you are concerned that any reminder that her breasts are fake will upset you. This may be a good reason for her to not get implants. Or she may just need to find a really good surgeon to make her look the best.

7

Why Does She Want Implants?

After interviewing several men whose women got breast implants, every man agreed on one thing – knowing WHY she wants implants is the most important part of breast augmentation.

There are many reasons your lady might be interested in getting a new set of breasts. While I can't be certain, you should feel confident that it has little to nothing to do with you.

Read that again. Her desire for breast implants most likely has nothing to do with you. Get over yourself.

No matter what, you will have to talk to your woman to find out what is the most important reason she wants to inflate her love bubbles.

Feelings of Inferiority

If you haven't figured it out yet, women are emotional creatures. The way your woman feels is more important to her than any fact. Has she ever said she "felt fat" in a pair of jeans, even though you knew damn well that she looked hot?

You will never fully understand all of her emotions. Accept that fact. Even she doesn't understand them all. But what you can understand is that "how she feels" is oftentimes more important than what you say, what you think, or what anyone else tells her.

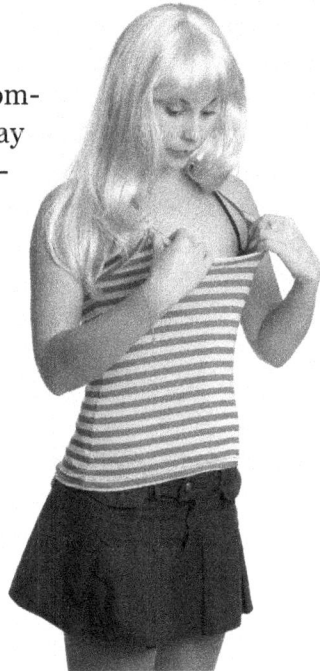

> Some women dye their hair because they think they look more attractive in a different shade. Women wear eye shadow, mascara, and lipstick because it makes them feel good and improves the way they present themselves to the world. Women want breast augmentation for the same reason: it makes them feel better about the way they look.
>
> *Dr. Vip Says...*
>
> Since late adolescence, when your lady friend realized that her chest was finished growing, she has wanted bigger breasts. That's it. That's the reason. She sees her friends, family, and many other women with bigger breasts, and when she looks at her own, she wants them for herself. And there's nothing wrong with that.

This is often the case with breasts. You've been programmed to like boobs by nature and by our society's constant focus on breasts. Go figure that women are similarly programmed to want big breasts.

If your woman has told you that she wants a boob job, chances are that she has felt like she doesn't measure up for a long time. Even if her boobs are perfect in your eyes, something in her head makes her think that she is inferior.

Maybe your lady has always had a large-breasted friend that always got more attention than she did. It could be that her little sister grew bigger boobs and that your woman felt like she lost the gene lottery. Maybe it's just all the movies she's watched that show the bra busters of Scarlett Johansson and the like.

As one researcher found, breast implants may make your woman feel like she has "gained something lost in early puberty"[1] as she catches up to others who grew more womanly when she didn't.

Because of these feelings of inferiority, most women with small breasts have used some product or technique to make their boobs look bigger at some point.

---

1 Gifford, S. Emotional attitudes toward cosmetic breast surgery: Loss and restitution of the "ideal" self. In Godwyn R., ed. Plastic Surgery and Reconstructive Surgery of the Breast. Boston: Little, Brown, 1976; 117.

Many women stuffed their bras with tissue paper in high school or used rubber inserts to make their breasts look bigger. Padded bras have been around for years, and some newer models have special pockets filled with water or gel so that they move more like natural breast tissue. You can even find videos on YouTube™ that show how a girl can use make-up in a special way so that it looks like she has more cleavage.

No matter what, if a woman is presenting herself as having larger breasts than she really has, she knows that she's being a bit deceptive.

This never hits home more than the first time she takes off her bra in front of a new guy. She expects to see the letdown in his face as taking off the bra makes what looked like average boobs disappear into a flat chest.

This feeling of letting a man down haunts many flat-chested women

This feeling of letting a man down haunts many flat-chested women, and it is not just the first time she takes off her bra, either. The 2nd time, 3rd time, the 20th time, the 100th time—every time she feels bad about letting him down. And this makes her feel even more inferior.

Then again, it may even be PARTLY your fault she wants implants (even if you never consciously did anything to suggest it). If you ever blatantly check out large-chested women in front of her, the message gets sent pretty quickly that you like large boobs. Maybe she's found "bigtits.com" in your internet browser history, or saw a copy of "Busty" in your car. She knows you like boobs.

The bottom line is that any woman who is thinking about getting implants thinks something about her breasts just isn't right. This can be the case with a woman of any age. Women who are already mothers tend to have other reasons for wanting breast surgery. But if your lady is young and not a mother, this is likely her main reason.

Feel Younger and Sexy Again

If your woman has been so kind as to provide you with several years of companionship and/or a few happy children, chances are she's not quite as hot as she used to be. Even if she takes great care of it, time and kids can really ravage a woman's body.

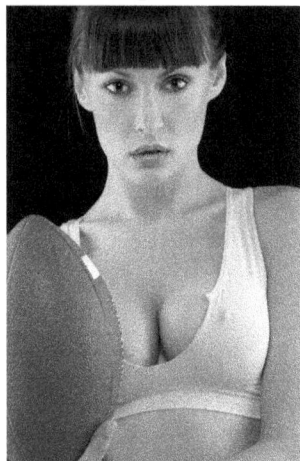

You may notice one little thing about your woman that makes her seem just 1$^{\%}$ less hot than she was when you first met. If you can see even one thing, then she can see 20 things that make her 90% less hot than she was then. Many women are their own worst critics.

To counteract the changes time has made, many women seek to look and feel younger. New perky breasts can make a woman of any age feel like a teenager again. They can attract attention that she hasn't had for a long time.

Wanting implants to feel young and sexy again is especially common amongst women in their 30s or older. If she's in that age range or has noticeably gotten less hot (for any reason), this is probably why your woman wants to upgrade her boobs.

Uneven Twins

Few women have perfectly even breasts. Very few. You may not be able to notice, but if you ask her, your woman will likely be able to tell you in a millisecond how her boobs are different.

There are many ways in which her breasts can be asymmetrical. She may have one that hangs a little lower than the other, or sits a little further out, or points in a different direction. Or one could just be smaller than the other.

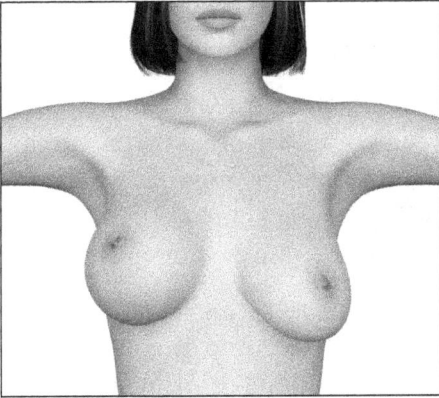

To a certain degree, a doctor can balance out uneven breasts. In some case these they can do this with different sized or differently-filled implants. However, implants could just increase the extent of any unevenness. In this case, her surgeon may choose to combine the augmentation with a breast lift or partial breast reduction.

If your lady sees her girls as uneven, this can lead her to want an upgrade.

Too Saggy

Some women have naturally saggy boobs. It's just how their breasts are. One of Jane's friends (who is a model) has fairly big boobs, but they hang down really far when her bra comes off.

Some women who started with perky breasts may find that "the girls" have headed toward their waists with age.

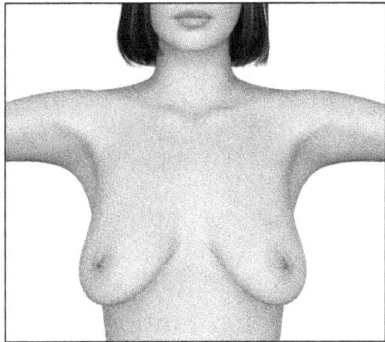

Whether it is due to the ravages of time and lifestyle, or the results of breast-feeding a child, many women lose breast volume with age.

Some experience a significant drop in breast height, and an unfortunate few are left with little more than small, empty bags of skin.

If your kids have "eaten away" your woman's boobs, she may cite this as the reason she wants implants.

Oftentimes to fix the sagginess, the surgeon will also perform another procedure known as a "breast lift". Breast lifts can create much perkier breasts by moving where the nipple is on the breast and removing some skin, but often result in more noticeable scarring. Many women feel that the trade off is worth it.

Again, you will have to talk with her and the surgeon to ensure that she has proper expectations prior to surgery.

Breast Cancer

If your woman has battled or is battling breast cancer, and had or needs to have a lumpectomy, quadrantectomy, or mastectomy, I offer you my deepest sympathies. Cancer and its treatment can wreak havoc on a body and make a woman feel incredibly unattractive.

Some women who must have breast tissue removed choose to live life without replacing what was lost. They may feel the lost breast is a badge of honor or reminder of what they survived.

Other women choose to have their breasts reconstructed so as to feel more womanly again. Getting breast implants as part of reconstruction can really help a woman feel more normal and bring back the spark to her personality.

If this is your reality, you should not be surprised that your strong lady wants breast implants after having her life thrown off-course by cancer. You don't have a defensible argument for wanting her to NOT get them.

Difficulty Finding Clothing That Looks Good

A lot of "sexy" clothes are made for women with at least moderately-sized breasts. That means swimsuits, tank tops, V-necks, and basically anything strapless (like a cocktail dress) can be downright embarrassing for a flat-chested woman to wear.

Chances are your woman has been frustrated on more than one occasion because she couldn't "fill out" a certain outfit like she wanted to. If she has always wanted to be married in a strapless wedding gown, breast augmentation may help her fulfill her dream of looking fabulous in the dress of her choosing.

If she gets bigger boobs, your woman will have different clothing options available to her. This desire may   be part of what is driving her to want implants.

While large breasts may help some women find clothes that fit more easily, many woman who get very large implants find it just as difficult to find clothes that fit their new sweater kittens. If clothing is partially motivating her, make sure she doesn't go too big.

Bad Reason Why!

Some women think that breast implants will solve all their problems. Breast augmentation can only enhance a woman's figure; it cannot solve any significant self-esteem issues and will not cause all of life's problems to disappear.

If your woman makes it sound like she is one of these "solve all my problems" women, you may need to help her face reality. Therapy may be the better option.

Why *You* Might Want Her to Go for It

As men, we are physiologically pre-programmed to like boobs. As noted anthropologist Desmond Morris taught in his book, *The Naked Ape*, breasts represent nourishment and power in primate society. For this reason, breasts represent female sexuality.

For the past few decades, the female sexual ideal of American culture has been one with large breasts. There is no question that they dominate our society. Look at clothes, advertising, movies, television, magazines, or cheerleaders' outfits. Blame Marilyn Monroe, Jayne Mansfield, and Dolly Parton.

Your woman is thinking about going for this touchdown because she has been taught that boobs are important. And to you and your animal brain, they are important!

On the other hand, you may feel like you are doing something wrong if you want her to get implants. You may feel like she's doing something "fake" or "unnatural".

What does it mean if you are with an "augmented woman" or a woman with "fake tits"? Is it "unnatural" and "wrong" like some people suggest?

What is natural? Droopy boobs? Small boobs? What about breast cancer? That's natural. Oh, and so is body hair. So is everything "natural" always so great?

Going to the gym, shaving her legs and armpits, and wearing make-up are all "artificial" but more socially acceptable ways that she makes herself look better.

She wants boobs. You instinctively want boobs and a happier woman. That's why you might want her to go for it!

Of course, there are many reasons you may be afraid or NOT want your lady to get breast implants. This book is to meant to help you understand why you might feel that way, inform you of the facts, and help you communicate your feelings if the facts don't make you accept her desire for augmentation.

* 8 *

What Is At Stake?

You now know what a boob job is and what its results might be, so you know what scoring a touchdown could be like.

But you probably want to know **what is at stake** in choosing to go for the touchdown. In a real football game, you could always end up fumbling or throwing an interception.

"Going for it" could be worse in the game of life than just "kneeling it" and keeping her real boobs.

Read that again. Breast implants may make things worse.

You need to know how you both might be affected.

First and foremost, breast augmentation is invasive surgery. There are several **health risks** that can cause women to worry.

Another thing that keeps many women from getting implants is the **cost**. Boob jobs are not cheap, and there are many additional expenses most people don't think about. The total cost can be much higher than expected. Some mothers feel guilty over the thought of spending money on themselves that could otherwise be spent on their children.

The **time investment** required for breast augmentation is off-putting to some women. In addition to the time it takes to find a doctor and have the surgery, there is a few-day intensive recovery period that she will need to probably

Boob jobs are not cheap, and there are many additional expenses most people don't think about.

take off from work. Also, breast augmentations can take up to a year to look really good.

Many men and women worry about how breast implants might affect their relationship. Some insecure men fear that with new breasts, and the confidence and new attention they bring, their women will leave them.

Other women hold back from getting implants because they worry that *people will think* less of them.

Finally, some women fear that breast implants might interfere with their daily activities, but that is unlikely.

Let's look at all these concerns in detail.

What are the Health Risks?

Football is a great game but players can be seriously injured. Guys get concussions, blow out knees, and pull hamstrings regularly. For instance, in the 2010 Preseason, Denver's Elvis Dumervil tore his pectoral muscle. He needed surgery and the recovery will keep him out the entire season.

Luckily, breast implants cannot result in any of these injuries, but there are some health risks to consider and be aware of.

Breast augmentation is a serious surgery, and any surgery creates the possibility of infection. Infections are rare, but

Risk	Likelihood[2]
Infection/Bleeding	1-2%
Nipple Sensation Loss	2%
Loss of Breast-Feeding	1%
Capsular Contracture	("unders") 1-18% ("overs") 18-50%

Most common breast augmentation health risks

---

2 Love, SM and Lindsey, K. Dr. Susan Love's Breast Book, 4th ed. Cambridge, MA: DaCapo. 2005. (p. 45 and 50)

any infection can spread and even cause death. Death is possible, but very, very, VERY rare in breast augmentation.

Anesthesia-Related Issues

With any major surgery, "going under" always carries the extremely small risk of not waking up.

Mothers and fathers usually worry about what happens to their children if mom doesn't wake up from the surgery or another complication occurs. Again, this is highly unlikely.

Surgeons almost always require a health exam (including blood work) prior to operating so that they can identify any special risk factors for the woman. It is very important for your woman to be completely honest with her surgeon about her health issues, concerns, and medications.

Your woman's anesthesiologist will also review all of this information later. His primary concern during the operation is monitoring your woman. He will look out for and prevent any complications.

If there's a health reason she should not have surgery, the doc will tell her so. If she goes through with surgery in spite of a doctor's warning, she may well be putting her life at risk.

If your woman has been honest with her surgeon and anesthesiologist, and they both deem her healthy enough to have the surgery, then she should easily handle anesthesia, and death should not be a concern.

Leaking Implants

Implants are silicone shells filled with either saline solution or silicone gel. Saline is nothing more than salt water and will not harm her in any way. So there's no reason to worry about leaking saline implants causing health issues.

Years ago, women shied away from silicone implants because they feared that the silicone filler material might leak and

> **Dr. Vip Says...**
>
> "Implant failure" is a rupturing of the implant. Like anything else, an implant will eventually wear out and need to be replaced. This can happen for any number of reasons, including trauma to the breast area. Also, the longer the implants are in place, the higher the risk of a rupture occurring.
>
> Saline rupture is very obvious—one breast will immediately look flatter. With silicone implants, rupture is noticed only on an MRI, which is the reason why an MRI is recommended every few years. Otherwise, the rupture may not be noticeable. While studies have shown no damage to the woman as a result of a silicone rupture, and that the silicone cannot "invade" other parts of the body, it is not recommended to leave a ruptured silicone implant in place.

cause health problems. This was when silicone filler was just a thick liquid (not a gel), before the FDA pulled them off the market in 1992.

In the years since then, implant makers have reformulated their silicone filler material. The silicone gel in these newer implants has stronger molecular cross-links than in the old ones, and these links help the implants better retain their shape and prevents them from leaking. The new cohesive silicone gel implants **will not leak** if ruptured.

If you go to YouTube™ and search for "Durability of Saline and Silicone Implants", you will find a video that shows what implants look like if they are poked with a needle or sliced with a scalpel. It even shows what happens when a cohesive silicone gel implant is sliced in half completely. Nothing leaks! It's like what happens when you bite a gummy bear in half.

The new cohesive silicone gel implants will not leak if ruptured.

These new silicone implants were approved by the FDA in 2006, but because they are still new, no one really knows how a silicone gel implant might behave if it were to rupture 20 years down the line.

When it comes to leaks, the health impact should be considered minor. The bigger concern with leaking implants is that another surgery likely will be needed to replace a leaking implant.

Loss of Sensation

For up to the first year post-op, some women claim their nipples are hypersensitive or the opposite—totally numb. Neither is very common, and most women who experience either return to normal sensation over time.

Usually, the sensation returns to normal, but there is a slight chance (<2%) that your woman may permanently lose some sensitivity to touch in her breasts.[3] This may be enough to turn some women completely off of the surgery.

Jane had an interesting experience. While her nipples were numb for several months following her surgery, they later regained sensation. And then got more and more sensitive. Eventually, her nipples were more responsive to my caresses and kisses than ever before!

Breast-Feeding After Implants

If your woman is thinking about having children in the future, there is a slight risk that she may not be able to breast feed them after an augmentation.

A common myth is that all women who get implants lose the ability to breast feed. In reality, it only happens in about 1% of breast augmentations. Of women getting breast reduction (a much more serious surgery), up to 50% can lose breast-feeding ability. But this isn't your woman.[4]

Some people fear that breast milk may be tainted in some way by implants. To the contrary, the FDA found that milk

3 Love (p.50)

4 Laursen, NH and Stukane, E. The Complete Book of Breast Care. New Yourk: Fawcett Columbine. 1996.

from women with silicone implants has no more silicone in it than that of non-augmented women.[5]

Complications

There are many complications that can develop after the surgery that have nothing to do with the surgeon's skill. Some are merely cosmetic, and may need to be surgically repaired (symmastia, ugly scars, bottoming out). Others can be serious health issues that may require immediate medical attention (hematoma, seroma, infections). You will discover more about these later.

Myths

There are many myths about breast implants that are completely untrue.

For years, people thought there was a connection between breast implants and connective tissue diseases (like arthritis) or autoimmune diseases, but dozens of scientific studies, covering thousands of women, have shown that **there is no connection**.

Similarly, research has shown that implants do not increase the likelihood of breast cancer.[6] This is a only a myth.

How Much Does Breast Augmentation Cost?

Just like when your team tries to bring in a big name free agent, you're going to have to spend some serious bucks if you want a good surgeon. Depending on where you live, expect to pay anywhere from $3,500 to $10,000 for a basic breast augmentation.

---

5 Gerber, D. and Czencko-Kuechel, M. 100 Questions and Answers About Plastic Surgery. Boston: Jones and Bartlett. 2005.

6 Love (p.52)

The total cost of the surgery and post-op purchases will likely be much larger!

The total cost may be $5,000 to $15,000!

Remember, find the best surgeon you can. It's well worth the extra money. Think not of it as an expense, but as an investment in her happiness and in the health of your relationship. On the other hand, higher price does not always equal better quality surgeon. Do your homework to find the right surgeon.

Health insurance usually does not cover breast augmentation. Some insurance carries may refuse to pay for future breast-related health issues, or may drop her coverage. Investigate this before choosing surgery.

Additional Surgery-Related Costs

There are many issues that can increase the overall cost of ownership of breast implants.

When choosing her surgeon, your woman will need to go on one or many consultations with prospective surgeons. Many surgeons will give free consultations, but others charge for their time. These consultations are usually in the $50-$100 range.

It's good to know that *silicone implants themselves cost about $1,000 more than saline implants*.

The FDA recommends women with silicone implants get an MRI 3 years after augmentation, and every two years thereafter to detect any ruptures. This might run you another $1200 or so every couple of years.

If the surgery went wrong or the implants just aren't sitting right in her breasts or she has developed a complication, there is a chance that your woman may need a revision of her surgery. A re-do may be needed as early as the first few weeks or months after the surgery. This is rather drastic and only happens in certain circumstances.

Some good surgeons are so confident in their work that they offer "free" re-dos, which would cost as little as the anesthesia and operating room fees. Other doctors (who are great surgeons too), choose to charge full price for any re-dos. Your woman should ask about this in her consultations and consider the answers when choosing a surgeon.

PAY ATTENTION:
Breast implants are NOT lifetime devices.

Even with a perfect surgery and recovery, your woman's implants **MAY** have to be replaced *after 10-20 years*. This is not always the case, but there is not ample data to guarantee otherwise. This is just the way it is, man, and means there may be even more money to spend down the road.

Of course, if your lady wants any other procedures to be performed (such as a breast lift or tummy tuck) at the same time as her boob job, there will be further expenses. And they won't be cheap!

New Wardrobe

One expense that your woman won't complain about is buying new clothes and bras!

After surgery, your woman is obviously going to need to throw away all her old bras and get new ones. This is probably about $100-$500 right off the bat, and may be more once the implants have "settled".

Much of modern fashion is made to showcase larger boobs. If your woman never had big boobs before, she probably never had certain styles of clothes (tops, dresses) that she really wanted. Now that she has boobs that will look good in such items, she may want rush out to get these clothes.

Be prepared for a big hit to your wallet. Depending on where she shops, clothing can run another $200-$2,000 (or $20,000 if she shops in Beverly Hills).

How Long Will it Take?

Breast implants are not an instant solution. This is major invasive surgery, and it will take a while for your woman's body to recover from the operation. It will also take months for her body to get used to the implants. Once it does though, they can be very nice.

Right after surgery, her boobs will be weird-looking. There's no way around that. For the first few weeks, they may look square-ish and sit high on her chest. HAVE FAITH! They will look better.

After a couple of months, "the girls" should round out and begin to drop a little as her body heals and adjusts to accept the implants. Seriously, a couple of months. Have patience.

By 6 months, most women's boobs will have dropped all the way to look more like natural breasts. It may take up to a year after the surgery before your woman's new breasts are fully settled. During this time, they will continue to get progressively softer and more jiggly.

You must have patience and NOT judge them too soon. The worst thing you can do is to get upset about them looking weird before they are ready.

Would you believe that some men are so insensitive as to

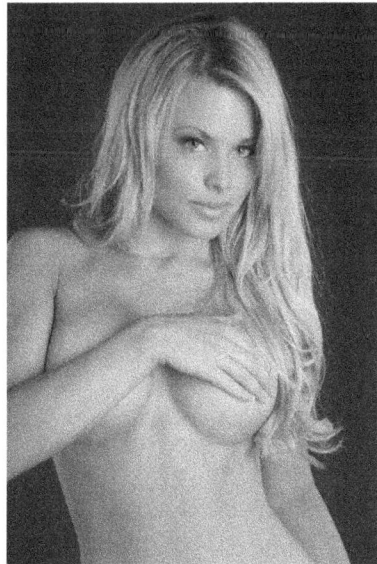

49

say mean things about their women's new breasts before they are ready?

DO NOT get mad at her or insult her. You will only hurt her self-esteem more and make her NOT want to have sex with you. This won't make either of you happy. You could easily ruin all the good things that the implants have done for her self-confidence.

It may take up to a year after the surgery before your woman's new breasts are fully settled.

When they are fully settled, your woman's breasts will hang more naturally as her muscles and breast tissue relax and the implant begins to "drop" down. They will develop more of a "fluffiness" that will make them seem more like natural breasts. Many people refer to this state of final settling as "dropped and fluffed" breasts.

Once your woman's breasts are "dropped and fluffed", you will be able to lift them up and squeeze them easily. Also, they will start to move and bounce more like real boobs (not "exactly" but "more like"). A more natural upper breast slope will develop, and her breasts won't sit up near her chin any longer.

How Might Implants Change Your Relationship?

Regardless of why your woman wants implants, getting new breasts will likely improve her self-image. She will hopefully have more self-confidence.

For some women, this makes them more outgoing and happier. They feel sexier and want to wear sexier clothing. After not being able to have sex in the initial post-op recovery stage, many women will find that their libido increases significantly the more they heal.

This can be the greatest thing for your relationship! If you've always been the horn dog in the relationship, her sex drive might actually catch up to (or surpass) yours. This can be a lot of fun for a while, but many women's libidos return to normal after the novelty of the new breasts wear off.

Other women may become more critical of themselves, finding other "flaws" that need to be "fixed". This complaining can be a downer and may strain your relationship. It can also affect your sex life if she doesn't like how she looks. ***This can be a big deal!! Watch out!!!*** Think about this carefully.

Regardless, if you work to help her throughout her breast augmentation decisions, surgery, and recovery, you will have ***invested greatly in your relationship***. The time you spend helping her can draw you closer together and help you understand one another better. It's not just about the new boobs. Going through the whole process together can change your relationship.

Could She Possibly Leave Me?

With all this new confidence in her body, you might be wondering if your woman will no longer think you are good enough for her.

Sure, some women are like a free-agent-to-be in a "contract year". They improve considerably right before they switch teams. However, most women just want the implants for the reasons discussed before.

There's no guarantee that your woman won't want to upgrade to another man once she's upgraded her looks. But if you have a strong relationship and help her through the process, it is unlikely.

No matter how your relationship is right now, you can make it a lot better by supporting her through the breast augmentation process. Help her make the decisions, and take care of her while she recovers.

This will bring the two of you closer together and will give you a bit more "ownership" in the new boobs (this has nothing to do with whether or not you paid for them). Even if she was planning to leave you, your involvement may rekindle interest in one another and could make her think twice before leaving.

Hopefully, her new confidence (and your confidence having her on your arm when you go out) will just make your relationship better.

What Others Think

Some women are hesitant to get implants out of fear what others may think about them. They especially worry about what their spouse, friends, parents, and children (current or future) will think of them.

This may bother you too. How long will it be before your buddies make jokes about you "sucking on plastic" (if you choose to tell them)? And what if your young daughter wants to get implants later on? What will you tell her? What is your mom going to think, and will she say anything bad to you about your woman?

Just as you cannot judge her breasts before they are ready, you can't let anyone else judge her for going through with the surgery.

There are many closed-minded people in this world who will look down on others for doing something they consider unnatural.

You may lose some people's respect if she chooses to go through with the augmentation. What's more important to you – how your woman feels or what some other people think about you and her? Consider this carefully.

Limited Activities

A few women are forward-thinking enough to realize that *very* large plastic implants in their chests may limit the activities in which they can participate. If your woman is very active in fitness activities that use a lot of upper-body strength (rock climbing, yoga, swimming), this worry may be holding her back. Also, if she is a runner, she might be concerned with how implants might affect the bouncing of her breasts while she jogs.

As child care can require significant physical activity, your woman may worry about how to deal with children if she cannot bend down or pick them up.

Women typically are only limited in their activities as they recover from augmentation. After a few weeks or months, your woman's surgeon will likely allow her to perform any activities she wants.

Thus, fears of limited activities should not prevent her boob job.

She Might Not Shut Up About It!

Even if everything goes well, and her new breasts are perfect, your woman might not shut up about them. This is just another part of the "cost" of the surgery.

The longer it takes for her breasts to "drop and fluff", the more likely it is she may complain. Keep her spirits up and

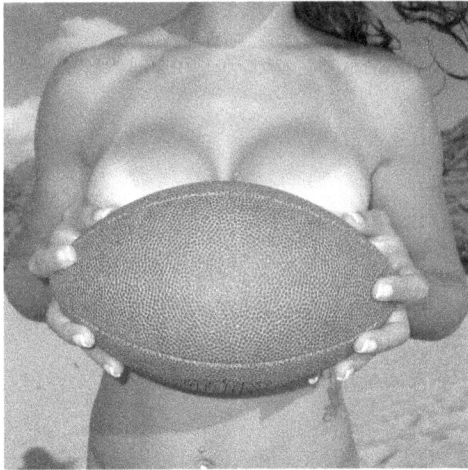

remind her that they will look good soon enough. Your patience will help her be patient.

Your woman may nit-pick and point out every little problem she sees with her breasts, or she could spend a lot of time bragging about them. No matter

what, be prepared to listen to her talk about them. Maybe your woman talks non-stop anyway, but at least now it's a topic you like, her knockers!

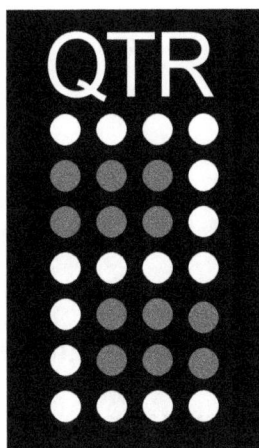

S<small>ECOND</small>

Q<small>UARTER</small>:

D<small>ECISIONS</small>

Questions This Section Answers:

How does she **decide to go for it or not?**

What are consultations and **why** does she need them?

How should she **choose a surgeon**?

How can she figure out what **she wants her new boobs to look like?**

How does she **communicate** this with the surgeon?

How **many choices** exist for breast augmentation?

What are the **"pros" and "cons"** of each of these options?

What do we do next once she's made her choices?

What can we do now to help her recovery later?

* 9 *

Kneel Or Go For It?: No Or Yes To Implants

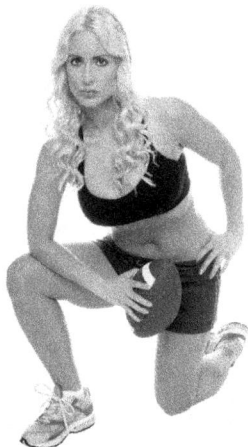

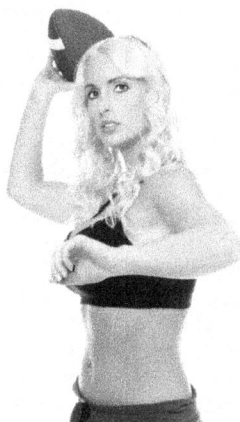

The timeout is nearly over...

It's time to make the decision...

Will she decide that your team should go for the touchdown or just kneel the ball? Will she get breast augmentation or not?

While it may be your money that will pay for the surgery, you have to remember one thing:

It. Is. Her. Body. She gets to decide.

You have to let go of the decisions. Follow her lead and give your opinion only when she asks for it.

I highly recommend that you tell her something along these lines: "Baby, I love you how you are right now, and I will continue to love you however you look after the surgery, should you choose to go for it. Do what is best for you."

She came to you to tell you that she is considering the surgery and now that you have both researched it, you can help her make the best decision.

How To Help Her Make The Decision

Unless your woman already had her mind made up before she came to talk to you, she likely wants your input for her decision whether or not to get a boob job.

To help her make the decision, you will need to talk to her. You should ask her what her opinion is and if she asks for it, give her your opinion.

Potential Pros	Potential Cons
Happier, More Confident Woman	Potential Health Risks
Better Looking Breasts	Costs $5,000-$15,000 Total
She Feels Sexier	Intense Recovery Period: Pain, Nausea, Swelling, Bed Rest
Potential Increased Libido	Complications Can Arise
Can Improve Your Relationship	She May Want to Leave You
She Can Wear Sexier Clothes	Takes Months to Look and Feel Good
Lots of Fun to Play With	Not Permanent: Revision or Replacement Likely Needed Later
Can Feel Very Natural	May Have Visible Scarring
Overcome Breast Tissue Loss from Age or Breast-Feeding	Slight Risk She Can't Breast Feed in the Future
Fix Unevenness	Other People Judge You Two
Other Men Jealous of You	Her Activities May Be Limited At First

Pros and Cons of breast augmentation

This is your woman, so you should know best how to talk to her. However, not all of us men are comfortable with having conversations about delicate subjects, especially when it comes to a subject that society has made awkward, like cosmetic surgery.

You should both understand and agree by now what her **main reason for wanting a boob job** is. Discuss how important this reason is to each of you and why.

On the other hand, you might disagree about which "pros" and which "cons" are most important to you. Any disagreement should spur further discussion. As long as you remember that this is her decision, and that your choice of "Pros" and "Cons" is just your perspective, you should be able to navigate this conversation like Barry Sanders through a weak defensive line—no problems at all.

Next, you should discuss how you two could get the "pros" without the "cons" of breast augmentation. Perhaps she'd be happier if she got a big new diamond ring or started going to therapy. Maybe a trip around the world would bring you closer together. See if there are any alternatives to surgery that are possible and desirable for you both. If you can get a happy woman without the risks of surgery, then it's win-win!

Be sure to discuss what you will do to minimize the possible impact of the "cons". If the scarring is something that worries you greatly, she can decide to look for a surgeon who has an excellent record of minimally-scarring breast augmentations.

...you should discuss where you will get the money or what you will give up to save money.

Next, you should discuss where you will get the money or what you will give up to save money. This part is not meant to be a downer. It's important that you understand what sacrifices will have to be made to get the benefits of the boob job. This will help you appreciate the great results even more.

Alternatively, if what you would have to give up for the surgery is more important to you, you may choose to delay or decide against the surgery. Finally, write down her final decision and whether or not you each find the benefits to be more valuable than the potential downsides.

This last part—the decision—may have to wait for a second, third, or twentieth conversation before it is finalized. Be patient, and let her make the decision at her own pace.

Talking Her Into Or Out Of Surgery

Do not do this. Do not try to do this. Do not try to make her change her mind once she has made her decision. You will fail, or worse, you will succeed in convincing her, but she will resent it for the rest of your relationship (which may not be too long).

On the other hand, if her decision is something that you feel will make it **absolutely impossible** for you to continue in your relationship, you may want to try convincing her one way or the other.

Let me reiterate that **this is unlikely to succeed,** but do what you must if you are in a desperate situation.".

* 10 *

Which Receiver?: Picking A Plastic Surgeon

In 1993, the late Reggie White became the first NFL player to be acquired as a free agent. Everyone knew how good he was, and lots of teams opened up their checkbooks to try to pay him as much as it took to get him on their roster.

Ultimately, the Packers won the rights to have him on their team. He went on to do great things for that team. He got 68.5 sacks while in Green Bay, setting the team record. He also led the defense to a Super Bowl XXXI victory. When he retired, he was the NFL's all-time sack leader and was inducted into the Hall of Fame on the first ballot.

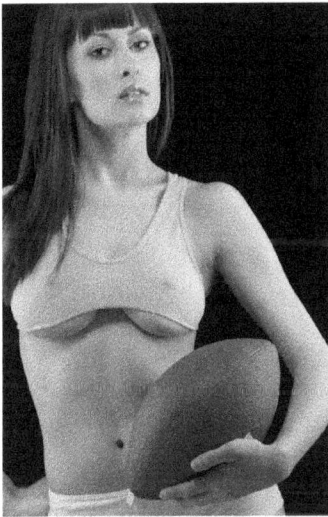

In 2010, free agency is a commonplace thing. Teams evaluate which veterans are on the market or will soon be on the market. They plan ahead, make room under the salary cap, and save up to be able to snatch up good players when they become available.

While it is possible to successfully throw a long pass to an average or poor wide receiver, the chances are not good it will succeed, especially if the opponents are strong.

Likewise, you may be able to get good breasts from an average surgeon, but the odds aren't good. Get the best surgeon you can afford. Picking the right surgeon can mean the difference between an amazing pair of breasts and years of regret.

I'll give you a simple process for finding the best surgeon:

- Start the List
- Narrow the List
- Pre-Consultation Prep
- Face-to-face Consultations
- Compare Surgeons
- Choose!

Starting Her List

Getting a Recommendation

Your lady may be able to avoid much of the process of searching for a surgeon by getting a recommendation for a great surgeon.

She could ask her friends, ladies at the hair salon, or doctors and nurses if they know of any really good surgeons. Obviously, if she knows anyone who has breast implants, that woman's opinion of should carry much more weight than others.

It's best to ask people that won't judge her and people whose opinions she really respects. If she wants to keep the surgery a secret, she might not want to ask anyone about it. In that case, she should...

Finding Nearby Surgeons

Without a great recommendation, she might need to just start with a search. Pull out the phone book and look under "Physicians-Plastic and Reconstructive Surgery" to find the plastic surgeons who practice in your area.

Or fire up the computer to do a Google search for "Plastic Surgery (Your ZIP code)", "Breast Augmentation (name of nearest big city)", "Breast Implants ...", or some variation thereof.

The Pros and Cons of Selecting
International Plastic Surgery

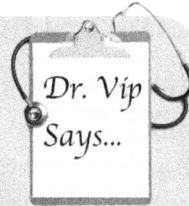

Dr. Vip Says...

You may have heard that going outside US borders, to Mexico or even farther away geographically, will save you money while delivering the same high quality of safety, care and results as those obtainable in the US. While this may be true in some instances, here are some things to think about:

- Will the savings on the procedure be used on travel expenses? Unless you are traveling alone, your trip expenses for airfare, meals and other items will be doubled.

- Will your health insurance cover your care if something goes terribly wrong?

- Does the licensing or accreditation authority in that country have the same standards for the operating room and plastic surgeon as we have here in the States? It's important to know that standards and procedural guidelines aren't identical everywhere in the world. While most Western European countries adhere to the same tightly-controlled regulations as the US, many former Soviet Bloc, third-world and Latin countries do not.

- What will you do about follow-up appointments months and years in the future?

- Who will treat you if you end up with a capsular contracture, rippling, uneven results or any of the other risks of breast augmentation?

- If you choose silicone implants, who will order the MRI every two years to make sure they have no leaks or ruptures?

- Who performs the anesthesia in an overseas procedure? An anesthesiologist? Can you confirm their accreditation and experience?

- Is the surgeon a member of a known and respected aesthetic society? Can you confirm the number (if any) of lawsuits or problems that surgeon may have had in the past with other patients?

Having a relationship with a reliable plastic surgeon who knows you, knows the implants you had inserted, and cares for you on an ongoing basis is well worth the money you will save by going overseas. And who knows, that relationship could also be a life-saving one.

Narrowing Her List

Now that she has a list to start with, she can start whittling it down. Ultimately, she will want to cut the list to a handful of doctors (say 2-5). That way, she can see multiple surgeons without going on too many consultations (which cost time and money).

Basic Online Researching

Each plastic surgeon is ultimately running a business, and the power of the internet for business is undeniable. Most plastic surgeons have some sort of website, but not all have very good websites. For every surgeon on your list, check out his website for a few things: overall look, reference to breast augmentation, board certification, professional association information, training information, before-and-after photos, and contact info.

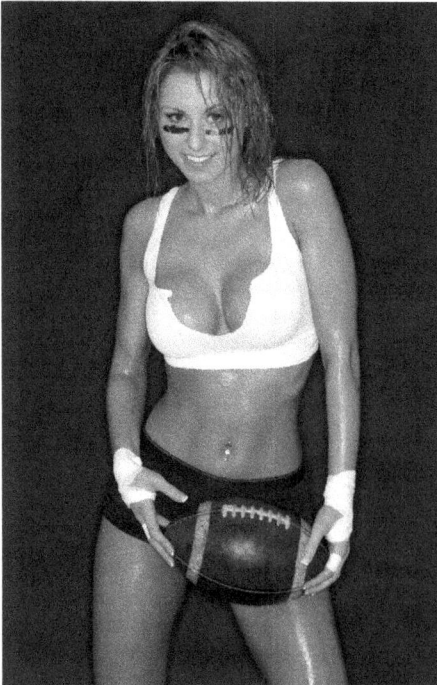

Overall, does the site look reputable? If it screams "quack!" or "cheapo!", you might want to strike that doctor from the list. Then again, he may just be "old school" and a phone call to his office might be the best way to learn about him (see next section).

Look on the web site to see if the doctor performs "breast augmentations" or "breast enhancement" or "breast implants". If you see no mention of it on his site, chances are that either he doesn't do augmentation at all or he does it very seldom, so he's not very good at it. Either way, if boob jobs are not on his website, cut him from your list.

Most surgeons who are proud of their work have some *before-and-after photos* displayed on their website. Take a quick peek to see if each doc on your list has pictures online. Browse through these for a few minutes, but don't get carried away as you still need to check out the other doctors' sites too.

On the site, look for the names of any boards he is certified by and any professional associations to which he belongs.

There are lots of "boards" that offer certification, but only one really matters: the American Board of Plastic Surgeons® (ABPS). This is the only plastic-surgery-related board recognized by the American Board of Medical Specialties.

Picking the right surgeon can mean the difference between an amazing pair of breasts and years of regret.

A doctor certified by the ABPS must go through years of specialized training and testing. While there is no guarantee that your woman will have a great surgical experience, an ABPS-certified surgeon is most likely to give her the result she seeks. Certification merely denotes training and does not promise competence in any technique or specific operation.

Some good surgeons may have extensive training but do not meet the requirements to be certified. If your woman meets with a doctor like this, she should be sure to ask him detailed questions about his training and past results.

For any other professional associations that the doctor links to, you can go to their webpages to see what they are all about. This may help sway you one way or the other on the doctor.

The most common question I get from prospective patients who call my office for information is "How much does a breast augmentation cost?" While financial concerns are understandable, please understand that calling before a consultation to ask about price isn't realistic. Every woman's body is different. A *good* surgeon must see the woman before giving a quote in order to understand if she needs a lift with her implants, or to explore any other concerns (scarring, previous breast surgery of another type, etc.) that could require extended time in the operating room.

Some offices will quote only the surgeon's fee over the phone, when in fact, the operating room and anesthesia fees must also be factored in to the final cost.

Remember, your woman isn't shopping for carpeting, which is roughly the same from store to store. She is shopping for the expertise and skill of a physician. It's a very different experience. The questions in the initial phone call should be focused on the surgeon's qualifications.

Dr. Vip Says...

Be sure to get all the correct *contact information* about the doctor.

Another great way to weed out the bad doctors and find great ones is to search through various online forums where women discuss their breast implant experiences. Online review sites such as "Yahoo!", "yelp!", and "CitySearch" can offer good information too. See the Resources section at the end of this book for more information.

Placing Pre-Consultation Calls

Because not all surgeons have good websites that easily list everything you need to know, the best way to trim your list is with phone calls.

There are a few questions you or she can ask in a short phone call to help you determine whether or not this doctor is worth the time and money of going in for a consultation.

Taking the few minutes to do this can save you a lot of time and hassle later on, and it will greatly increase your chances of finding the right plastic surgeon with ease.

Starting with her narrowed list, you or (more likely) she should call all the doctors and ask some basic questions. The best way to get these questions answered is to ask for the "Office Manager" or "Patient Coordinator", who tends to be more knowledgeable than the receptionist. It's best to call around 10 am if possible, since the manager is likely to be more fresh and isn't too busy yet with the hustle and bustle of the day.

Print out the free worksheet at
www.FootballAndBoobs.com/calls

Print it out, and ask the questions of each doctor's office you call. Based on these few questions, you can easily eliminate unqualified doctors from your search list.

From your calls, you will discover that some surgeons won't do breast augmentations, some will give a ballpark price estimate that's way out of your price range, and some might be just right for an in-person consult.

If the answers are satisfactory, she should schedule a face-to-face consultation with that surgeon.

Preparing for the Consultation

Once she has scheduled a few consultations, your woman should do some homework of her own to prepare. Before the consultation, she should be able to:

- Describe what she doesn't like about her breasts.
- Describe (or show with a picture) how she wants her breasts to look
- Find an example of the doctor's previous work that shows what she wants (if possible)
- Know which questions she will ask during the consultation
- Know what to look for during the consultation

What Does She Feel Is Wrong?

First, she should be able to clearly explain to you what it is that she doesn't like about her current breasts. You should not say to her, "Oh, but that doesn't matter!," thinking that you are supporting her natural beauty. You may make her feel like you think her feelings are invalid. Just let her say what she doesn't like, so she can practice for when she is talking to the doc. If you must say something, try "I can see how that could be important to you", after she points out a flaw.

What Does She Want?

Next, she should be able to explain what she wants her breasts to look like. The most *basic* thing is for her to pick a cup size that she wants, but that's not really good enough.

One thing you probably didn't know is that bra cup sizes are by no means standardized. Different brands and different styles within a single brand can fit very differently.

Sometimes Jane's bra is a C cup, other times it's a DD. So quoting a cup size doesn't really tell a surgeon exactly what she really wants.

She needs to be able to describe how she wants her breasts to look.

One way to do this is to look in magazines or online for photos of breasts. She should find a few examples of what she

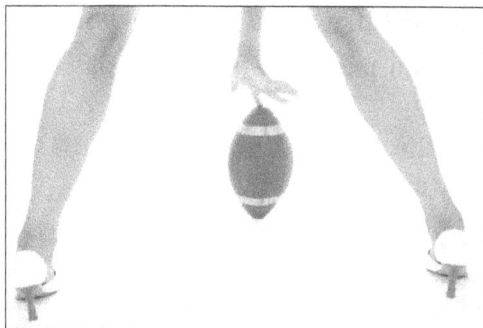

wants her breasts to look like, and print or tear them out and bring them to the consultations. (This is the part where you get to look at other women's boobies!)

While this part can

be fun, showing the doc a picture is not foolproof. Photos can be deceptive, and a doctor can't always tell what the models' real chest dimensions are. The pictures are simply to help him understand "the look" your woman wants.

The rest of your lady's body is the context for her future boobs. The breast size she's starting with may limit how big she can go. Her skin will only stretch so much, her chest is only so wide, and that means only so much implant can fit inside.

If she is not starting with very much (A-cup or smaller), her new boobs probably won't look very natural if she goes any larger than a C-cup (in some cases, a C may be too big too). Any bigger, and the chances they will look noticeably fake are substantial.

The most beautiful women in the world are well-balanced. If they have large chests, they have large butts too. Small, tight buns look best with small or medium-sized breasts.

A super skinny girl with no ass but a giant set of breasts often looks absurd. Girls that do this look like they are so top-heavy that the slightest breeze will tip them over, and everyone will know they have fake breasts.

Jane and her surgeon worked together to give her amazingly natural-looking breasts. But she knows a lot of women who really want the totally fake, "coconut" look. You two should talk about what will look best on your woman and the look she is going for.

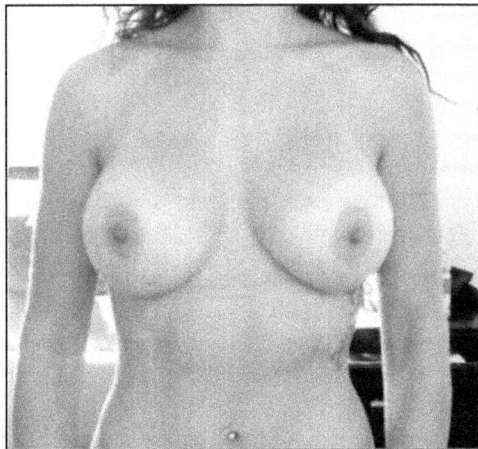

Jane's breasts look natural

69

How Good Is He?

Just like you'd review lots of video on a potential free agent wideout before you signed him, you should review examples of the work of each potential surgeon. Look through any of the "before and after" photos he has available online, or swing by his office to look at his book of photos. Even doctors with online albums usually have many more photos in the office.

Pay special attention to any photos where the "before" looks like your woman and the "after" looks like what she wants her breasts to look like. She will want to show this specific set of photos to the surgeon later. Keep in mind that because all women are built differently, he cannot guarantee that she will turn out like the woman in the photo.

Also, she should check out if any malpractice suits have been brought against him. You can do this by calling or visiting the website of your state's medical board. Literally searching "california medical board" brings you within two clicks of searching for a doctor by name. Not all states have such functionality, and you may need to call or email your state's board to find out about a particular surgeon.

She can also look for feedback from patients on the internet. Scrolling through certain online forums will yield a wealth of data on who is nice to patients, who does great

Your woman should investigate her potential surgeons with the state medical board. Are there any lawsuits against him? While it's not uncommon for even a great surgeon to have a lawsuit, a pattern of suits may suggest a problem.

Dr. Vip Says...

Have any of the surgeons on her list ever been brought in front of the medical board on charges of malpractice? Have any of them had their license suspended? These are things that often aren't publicly known but, believe me, she will want to know. Before and after photos are great, but in terms of safety and ability to deal with complications, she needs know more about her surgeon's history.

work, and who is just so-so. Check out the "Resources" section in the back of this book for a list of forums.

Getting Her Questions Ready

She should also know what questions she wants to ask the surgeon during each consultation. She can download the list at
www.FootballAndBoobs.com/consults
to get a list of useful questions. She should print multiple copies of her final list of questions and take them to each surgeon she consults with so that she can take notes.

Will You Go With Her?

Finally, you two should discuss whether or not she wants you to go with her to any of the consultations. She may want you to stay in the waiting room or she may want you to be by her side the whole time.

For some women, it's a relief to have her man there to support her. For others, it can be weird, as she will likely have to take her shirt off in front of another man.

Reassure yourself that it's okay for the surgeon to look at her breasts, because that is likely to happen. He may touch them too. That's the best way for him to determine the thickness of her skin and tissue to decide what will be best for her.

This might be a little awkward for you, but you should realize he's looking at her breasts like Adam Viniatieri studies the

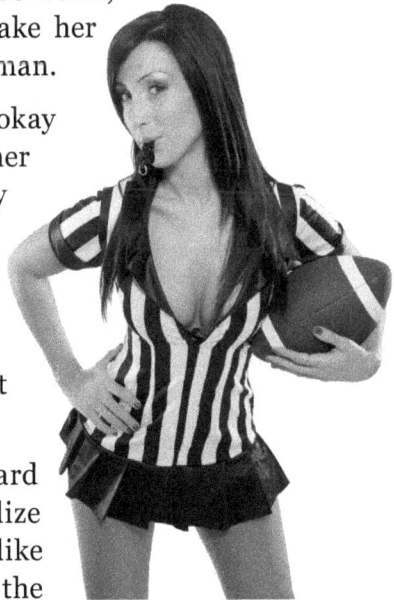

grass where he will plant his non-kicking foot before a big field goal.

If she wants you there, ensure she schedules her consults at times that work for you.

Also, be prepared to be completely ignored if you do go. Some doctors try to include the man through the whole consult, and some barely even acknowledge him until the very end. Discuss with your woman how much she wants you to talk if she wants you to go.

Dr. Vip Says...

During the consultation, the plastic surgeon will review the surgical procedure, its risks, benefits, and alternatives, review implant materials (saline vs. silicone), placement of the implant (submuscular vs. subglandular), types of incisions, pain control, infection, bleeding risks, types of anesthesia, dressings, recovery, time off, and any other potential complications.

The consultation is your lady's opportunity to meet the surgeon and his staff. Are they polite & kind? Do they seem genuinely concerned about her? Do they answer each of her questions thoroughly? Do they ask if she has any questions remaining at the conclusion of the consultation? Does she like them? Is she clear on pricing, what is included, and any additional costs? Be aware of all of these things, as well as the skill of the physician.

Ask lots of questions—bring a list of them that you both created at home from this book and from conversations with friends who have had implant surgery. Ask if the surgeon is a plastic surgeon and not simply a cosmetic surgeon—there's a big difference. Ask if the surgeon is board eligible or board certified in plastic surgery by the American Board of Plastic Surgery. A surgeon can be board certified in anything, including OB/GYN, family medicine, emergency medicine, etc., but not be a board certified plastic surgeon. Further, board certification does not guarantee competency.

Be clear when you visit each surgeon's office—tell them you're visiting with a handful of surgeons to gather all the information and will then make a decision, so they know you aren't going to be ready to make a decision right away. Beware of offices that pressure both of you with sales tactics such as a "today only" discount or any other benefit that wouldn't be available should she put off her decision

Meeting Surgeons Face-to-Face

Any time a team is considering signing a free agent, they not only watch game tape but they also bring him in to meet him in person, to get to know him a little and to see how he might fit in with the team.

As we discussed before, picking the right surgeon is the most important decision in the whole boob job process. Face-to-face consultations are the best way for her to pick the right surgeon.

The following are what your woman should try to get out of any consultation she goes on:

- Establish rapport between her and the surgeon
- Share her goals with the surgeon
- Learn what the surgeon suggests is best for her
- Surgeon explains the procedure and recovery in detail
- See examples of the surgeon's work
- Surgeon answers all her questions (including price)
- Surgeon examines and may measure her breasts

It has been said that the consultation with a surgeon can be like a cross between a test drive and a blind date. It can be a little awkward for both her and the surgeon (and you too, if you attend). It's normal for her to feel nervous about revealing her flaws to a stranger and having him scrutinize them. Reassure her that it's okay.

> To maximize your helpfulness to your woman, keep track of all of the information that you receive, and take detailed notes when you visit each office. How does each surgeon answer each question? Make sure you write down the answers to each of your questions for later comparison. Once you leave the office, evaluate the pros and cons of that practice before you forget. This way you can sit down later in a calm, stress-free environment, and make a final choice. He will then likely explain what the procedure and her recovery will be like.
>
> *Dr. Vip Says...*

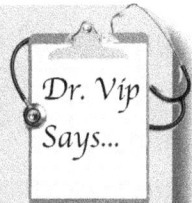

The primary purpose of the consultation is to give your woman an opportunity to get to know the doctor and his staff. She has to be comfortable with them. She will put a lot of faith into their ability to take care of her, so she needs to be able to trust them.

If she is really uncomfortable with a certain surgeon or his staff (how nice they are, how much time they spend with her, or how the office looks), remind her that it's okay to take that one off the list. You don't want a "clubhouse cancer" on your little team.

The second major purpose of the consult is for the doctor to learn what she is looking for in her new boobs. He will ask her what she doesn't like about her boobs to better understand what she wants and expects. She will tell him the size and amount of cleavage she would like, and her opinions on scar locations and which implant material she'd prefer. It helps if she has photos to show what she wants. This is where her preparation will pay off.

After explaining her desires, she will take off her top and the doc will study what her current boobs and rib cage are like. He may touch or just look.

Based on her anatomy and his personal preferences, the doctor will tell her what he would do to help her achieve her goals. He might give her options or simply tell her outright which of the detailed choices he thinks she needs. Most doctors will suggest a certain implant type, size, insertion location, and placement.

Looking at more photos will give a more complete picture of how good he is.

He might even have her try on "sizers" to help her understand how different size implants might look on her.

She can record the doctors' suggestions on the consults worksheet she printed. Or if you are there, it might be easier for you to write it all down.

If you two didn't do it online already, she should ask to see some examples of his previous work during the consultation. Since most doctors just like to show examples of their best work, she should ask to see each surgeon's complete portfolio.

Looking at more photos will give a more complete picture of how good he is. It also increases the chances that your lady will find another woman whose chest "before" looks like hers does now, so she can get a better idea what her results might be from that surgeon.

If the doc only has a physical picture book and she really likes a certain set, maybe she can snap a pic of the good before and after shots with her camera or phone. These can help later when comparing surgeons. She may need to be a bit sneaky about taking the photos.

In addition to photo proof, she may want to hear what kind of experience other girls have had with the surgeon. She can ask the office staff for a list of referrals. Another sneaky way is for her to make the best of her time in the waiting room by asking the women there what they think of that surgeon. Some of the women have probably had an operation and are back for follow-up appointments.

The final purpose of the consultation is for her to ask the doctor some questions. From his credentials and experience, to where he performs his surgeries, to his revision surgery policy, and to what she can expect in recovery, she should ask him as many questions as she needs to in order to feel comfortable with him operating on her.

Plastic surgeons are required to perform their procedures in certified, qualified facilities that have been built to specific standards so that they are capable of addressing most complications. If you have any questions about the facility where your girl will have her implants inserted, ask to see the certification, licensure and/or accreditation information.

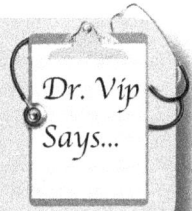

Dr. Vip Says...

Again, there are some great consultation questions for her to choose from available at

www.FootballAndBoobs.com/consults

The doctor may give her a narrower price range based on what he suggests. Very few doctors give a flat rate for any surgery, and most will give a different price depending on each woman's situation. She should ask for a quote if he doesn't offer it.

Lather, Rinse, Repeat

Even if she is convinced that the very first doctor she saw was perfect for her, she should go consult with another doctor (if for no other reason than to convince her how perfect doctor #1 is).

Getting consultations with multiple surgeons is the best way to find the one that she likes the best. I know this may be annoying, but you need the right surgeon.

As mentioned before, some surgeons will give a free consultation, but others can charge quite a pretty penny for it. Some run as high as $500, but most docs that do charge are between $50 and $100. Usually this charge is later deducted from the price of the surgery. Surgeons who require this fee do so to prevent your woman from skipping the scheduled consultation, and wasting everyone's time.

However, the consultation price won't really tell you how good the doc is. They charge the price people are willing to pay. Each surgeon is, after all, running a business.

It's important to be choosy about the surgeon who will sculpt your woman's new body. If you are buying a car, every state has a "lemon law" if you end up with a dud. Unfortunately, there are no "lemon laws" for breast implants. If you make the wrong choice in surgeon, you are unfortunately stuck with the results because you obviously can't return the breast implants. Therefore, keep in mind caveat emptor—buyer beware.

Dr. Vip Says...

In terms of consultations with surgeons, consider visiting with at most, three surgeons. More than three create too much confusion when it comes to making a final decision.

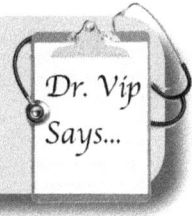

Dr. Vip Says...

The money can make getting consults fairly costly, but it is worth it. Paying $150 to realize that Dr. Meanguy won't be nice and won't be able to give her the breasts she wants could save you thousands of dollars and unnecessary stress!

Helping Her Pick the Surgeon

Based on how the consultations go, pick a surgeon. She can just go with the surgeon that made her feel the best, or you two can sit down and do all the math to see which will be the least expensive. Figure out which one meets all of her needs the best.

You should weigh all the options from the doctors she saw, and do what feels best. If no one seems right, she should be willing to wait and look more.

If she is having trouble choosing a surgeon, you can download the worksheet at
        www.FootballAndBoobs.com/surgeon
It will help you compare all the surgeons fairly and choose the best doctor for her.

11

Picking the Play: Decisions

After picking the surgeon, making all the detailed choices is next most important. Unfortunately, many of these decisions are linked, so when you choose one, you might limit what you can do with another choice.

The right surgeon will guide your woman through the detailed choices by telling her what he thinks will best to help her achieve her goals. However, because of personal preferences or surgical experience, some doctors suggest things that may not be in her best interests. That's why it helps for the two of you to know what the choices are.

In this chapter, you'll find a brief overview of the options she may have. This section is not meant to be comprehensive, but will give you enough knowledge to understand what the options are and which decisions she is rambling about.

Implant Material	Saline	Silicone
Implant Position	Above Muscle	Below Muscle
Incision Site	Above the Fold	Around Areola
	Armpit	Belly Button
Implant Volume	How Big? How Many CCs?	
Implant Profile	Moderate, Moderate Plus, or High (a.k.a. Low, Moderate, or High)	
Implant Shape	Round	Teardrop (a.k.a. Anatomical)
Implant Surface	Smooth	Textured

Major breast augmentation choices

Your lady may get overwhelmed with the number of decisions to make, and your helping her make those decisions could improve your relationship.

As long as your lady is willing to let you help her, do it. But never forget that these are ultimately her decisions and she is the one who will have to live with the results.

She and the surgeon will discuss these decisions in detail when she goes in for her final pre-operation (pre-op) appointment.

Silicone vs. Saline

The type of implant you choose will dictate a lot about the boob job and how your woman's new breasts turn out. She will have to choose between silicone and saline implants.

Silicone Implants

Silicone implants feel more like natural breast tissue, and usually cost about $1,000 more than a similarly sized set of saline implants.[7]

Also, silicone implants are inserted into the body pre-filled. This means the incisions must be big enough for the filled implant to fit through. Thus, a silicone implant needs a bigger incision compared to the same size saline implant. Bigger cuts mean bigger scars.

Inserting the implants pre-filled also means that the surgeon is limited as to where on her body he can make the incisions. Silicone implants are usually inserted through an incision around the areola, through an incision slightly above the "crease" on the bottom of her breast, or through her armpit.

Years ago, there were some suspicions that older versions of silicone implants caused health problems. Although no conclusive evidence linked the implants to any diseases or health complications, they were pulled off the market in 1992.

However, the manufacturers went back to the drawing board and overhauled the technology used in silicone im-

7 Loftus, JM. The Smart Woman's Guide to Plastic Surgery, 2 ed. New York: McGraw-Hill. 2008. (p. 127)

As of late 2010, the FDA is studying "new and improved" silicone implants, dubbed "gummy bear" implants. They are still pending FDA approval, but can be used by doctors approved to use them in specific situations. They are scheduled to be approved soon, but as of this writing, we're still waiting.

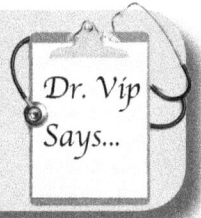

Dr. Vip Says...

plants. Newer implants are much less likely to rupture, and the filling inside does not run and is more cohesive (due to stronger molecular cross-linkings), so it will stay put even if a rupture does occur.

The FDA approved the use of cohesive silicone gel breast implants in November 2006 (after a 14-year ban and over a decade of testing).

The FDA recommends that any woman with silicone gel implants get an MRI of her implants taken three years after her surgery and every two years thereafter to detect any possible rupture. This is not required, but it is strongly recommended.

Another consideration that may come into play is that the FDA does not allow silicone implants to be put into women younger than 22. However, some doctors are willing to bend this rule.

Finally, since silicone gel implants have only recently been put on the market, the long-term effects of a rupture and how the implants hold up after 15 or 20 years is unknown.

Silicone implants have a lot going for them, but they may not be right for your woman. Her other option is saline.

Saline Implants

Saline implants don't feel as real as silicone, but they are less expensive and offer one huge advantage: flexibility.

Saline implants are inserted empty and then filled up once inside the breast pocket. This means they can be put in

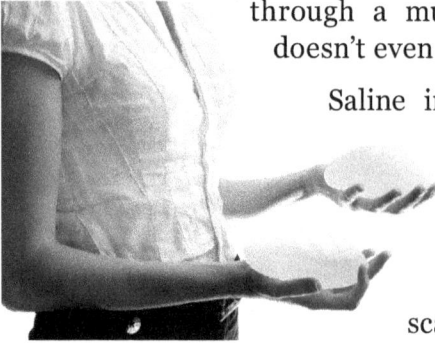

through a much smaller hole, which doesn't even have to be on the breast.

Saline implants can be inserted through the belly button or through the armpit. Yes, you read that right. The belly button! This keeps the scars off the boobs and hidden from view.

Saline implants are also flexible in that the doctor can fill them up a little extra as is necessary during surgery. Each implant can be filled a little bit differently to help even out her breasts (to an extent).

The downside of saline implants is that they can make breasts feel more artificial.

The chances are that you **will be able to feel the implant** are higher, and that might bug you or her. The least natural-feeling combination is when a woman starts with very little breast tissue (A-cup or smaller) and gets very large saline implants "over the muscle" (as described later).

The larger the implant, the more it stretches her skin, and the thinner the skin and breast tissue are spread. That means there's less boob to shield your eyes and grubby paws from the implant. Large saline implants with little breast tissue to cover them are likely to to easily felt and show ripples, which may bother you or her.

The downside of saline implants is that they can make breasts feel more artificial.

Choosing the Implant Type

The decision is between the flexibility and safety of saline and the realistic feel of silicone gel implants. Either one can be a great decision. A surgeon's suggestions on saline versus silicone can be important, but it is important that your lady knows what she really wants (and that you agree with her decision).

Saline Implants	Silicone Implants
Feel less natural	Feel more realistic
Show ripples more	More expensive
Smaller incisions	Usually bigger scars
More options for incision locations	Incisions on or near breasts
Easy to notice if rupture occurs	Suggested MRIs to check for ruptures
Can be filled differently to even out breasts somewhat	Safety in case of rupture not 100% known

Implant Position

There is no place within the breast that is naturally made for implants. The two most common places that the implant can be placed are "over" the pectoral muscle or "under" it.

With "overs" (technically called "sub-glandular augmentation"), the breast tissue is separated from the pectoral muscles so that the implant sits on top of the membrane (a.k.a. fascia) that covers her pectoral muscles but under her mammary gland.

"Overs" Sub-Glandular Breast Augmentation	"Unders" Sub-Muscular Breast Augmentation
Nipple Pectoral Muscle Implant Fatty Breast Tissue	Pectoral Muscle Ribs Implant Mammary Glands
Heals Faster	Longer Healing Process- Muscles Must Stretch
Better with Silicone	Good for Saline or Silicone
Can Show Implant if Little Breast Tissue to Start With	Hides Implant Better if Little Breast Tissue to Start With
Little Movement	Implant May Move When Pectorals Flexed

Breast implant position options
(Modified from image source[8])

"Overs" are best for girls with more breast tissue to start with or who have a little bit of sag to their boobs. If your lady has a lot of breast tissue to start with, she can look really natural with "overs", but if she has very little to start with, they may look more fake this way. If she chooses to go "over" the muscle, silicone implants may be better as they generally look and feel better than salines.

The other most common placement of breast implants is under the pectoral muscle. In "partial sub-muscular augmentation" or "unders", the pectoralis majoris muscles are lifted up and the implants go under the pecs.

---

8 http://www.fda.gov/cdrh/breastimplants/labeling/inamed_patient_labeling_5900.html

Surgeons typically recommend "unders" for women with little breast tissue. Since the muscle covers the upper edge of the implant, "unders" provide a more natural slope. This technique makes the new boobs look a lot more natural for girls who don't have a lot to start with.

This implant placement takes longer to heal and to look good because the pectoral muscles have to stretch and adjust to having implants underneath them.

Jane got her implants under the muscle. She had difficulty in the first few days after the surgery any time she tried to move her arms because her pec muscles were not happy about the intruders underneath. After about six months, her muscles had completely adjusted and she was able to resume all her activities.

Sometimes when she flexes her pecs picking something up, her whole boob moves. It's no big deal (and sometimes kinda funny), but you or your woman may be creeped out if this happened to your girl.

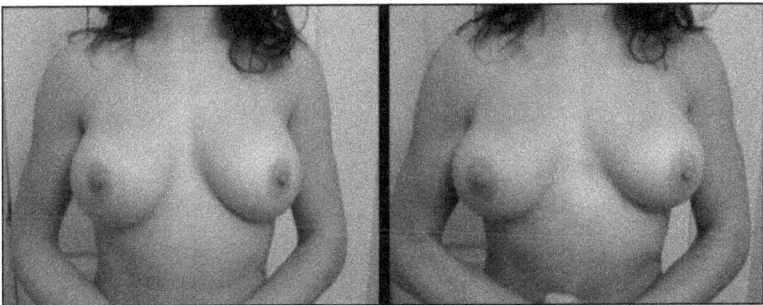

Not Flexing   **Flexing Hard**

Some doctors think the muscle movement muscle can cause "unders" to slowly migrate towards the sides, causing a loss of cleavage.

"Overs" vs. "Unders" should be decided by your girl and her surgeon.

Some surgeons use a third, relatively new placement, in which the implant is placed above the pectoral muscle but below the fibrous membrane or fascia that covers the muscle. This "subfascial" placement offers support for the implant from the fascia but avoids the displacement that muscle activity may cause because the implants are outside the muscle.

Since this is a relatively new procedure, not many surgeons are proficient in it. If a surgeon suggests this for your woman, ask to see several examples of work he's done this way.

Incision Sites

In order to insert breast implants, the doctor must make an incision on your woman's body. There are only so many places the cut can be made, but there are more than most men expect.

There are trade-offs for possible incision point. Read on to learn what each one means about where her scars will be.

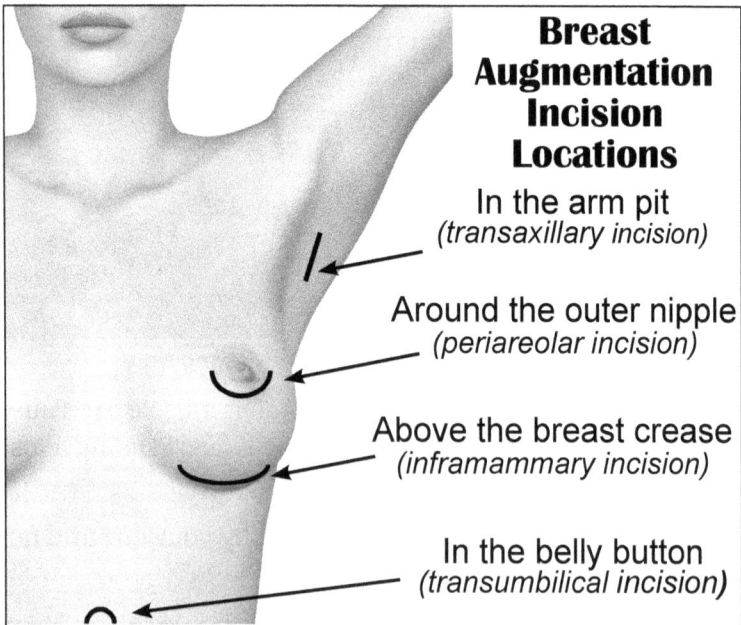

Breast Augmentation Incision Locations

In the arm pit
(transaxillary incision)

Around the outer nipple
(periareolar incision)

Above the breast crease
(inframammary incision)

In the belly button
(transumbilical incision)

Above the Breast Crease

When surgeons first started giving women breast implants, they put them in through the most logical spot—under the breast above the fold where her boob meets her chest. This type of augmentation is technically called "inframammary", but is more frequently called things like "under the breast", "in the crease", or "above the breast fold". Some of these names can be deceiving because technically, the incision is just a bit above the crease.

This incision site gives the surgeon the best access to the breast and makes it easiest to insert large silicone implants. This usually creates a scar about 1-2.5 inches long that could be visible when topless. However, when the breasts fully heal and "drop", the scar is usually hidden in the fold.

If you think it would bother you to see her implant scars when you are going down on your lady or when she does nude jumping jacks (how often is that?), then this incision site might not be the best for her. Discuss this.

Around the Areola

A lot of women don't want a line under each boob that might show when they wear a bikini. Surgeons have developed a technique in which they cut a semi-circle around the edge of her areola (the dark area around the nipple) and use this hole to insert the implant. In doctor-speak, this is called a "periareolar" incision.

This technique can leave a scar around the edge of the areola. Usually, this scar is not very noticeable due to the difference in skin tone between the areola and breast skin, but sometimes it can be quite apparent. If she chooses this incision, scarring can be an issue. Make sure that she chooses a highly experienced surgeon by studying his previous work photos. Remember to take into account how your woman scars.

Either silicone or saline implants can be inserted with a periareolar incision, provided her areola is big enough in diameter.

Remember, silicone implants are filled before they are inserted, so if your lady has a small areola and wants really big silicone implants, this may not work. They may just be too big for the hole. The surgeon will know this and likely will suggest an alternate incision spot or smaller implant.

Armpit and Belly Button

Surgeons understand that women want breast implants to make their boobs look better, and that scars on her breasts are not really "better looking". Smart doctors have developed techniques to hide augmentation scars by inserting the implant through incisions that are not even on the breast. They use not-so-obvious places like the armpit or the inside of the belly button.

Operations where the surgeon goes in through the armpit are known as "transaxillary breast augmentations" or "transax" for short. Belly-button surgeries are technically called "transumbilical breast augmentations" or "TUBA".

Transax and TUBA operations can be very tricky, and if your woman wants either of these, she MUST find a doctor that specializes in that incision type.

One advantage of the "transax" is that in some cases, silicone implants (usually less than 400 CCs) can go in through the armpit too. But since the armpit is far from the sternum, it can be difficult for the surgeon to create good cleavage. A slight disadvantage is that the armpit scar may be visible when your woman has her arms in the air (dancing, playing volleyball, picking up a child).

Since the belly button is even farther away, the implants must travel further under the skin for a TUBA than for a transax augmentation. The doctor must make "tunnels" under the skin to make this possible by pulling the skin away from the muscles. This results in sore abdominal muscles for several days after the surgery.

On the plus side, everyone's belly button is just one big scar anyway, so another scar there usually isn't too noticeable. You won't find the scar unless you are REALLY looking for it, especially if she has an "innie".

Jane got her saline implants put in through her belly button (TUBA), and the incision scar is amazing. You really cannot tell there was a cut there at all. She felt the extra pain was really worth the lack of scars and was a great decision.

Incision Decision

On the next page, you'll find a table summarizing the "pros" and "cons" of each incision site and what types of implants can be used with each site.

It's important to listen to what the surgeon thinks is best to achieve the look your woman wants. But if your lady has a certain incision location in mind, this might drive your choice of surgeon.

It's important to listen to what the surgeon thinks is best to achieve the look your woman wants.

For instance, Jane really wanted the belly button augmentation, and ruled out any surgeons that couldn't perform that a TUBA. She was able to be this picky because she was living in a city where there are many plastic surgeons. If your woman is not so lucky, she may need to travel to find her ideal surgeon.

Breast augmentation incision location choices

	Inframammary (crease)	Periareolar (nipple)	Transax (armpit)	TUBA (belly button)
Implant Types	Any Implant	Most Implants	All Saline and Small Silicone	Saline Only
Pros	Best access for Surgeon Most Surgeons Can Perform	Good Access Scar Less Visible Most Surgeons Can Perform	No Scar on Breast	No Noticeable Scar Least Traumatic to the Breast Tissue and Nipples
Cons	Most Visible Scar Scar Visible from Below and Possibly from Under Bikini Top	Possibly Noticeable Scar Slightly Higher Likelihood of Nipple Sensation Loss	Possibly Visible Scar in Arm Pit Limited Silicone Implant Sizes Possible Not All Surgeons Can Perform	Not for Silicone Implants Abdomen Painful for a Few Days Few Surgeons Can Perform

Implant Volume

Implant sizes are much more complicated than you would think. It's not as easy as "Give her a C-cup". Two girls can start with the same bra size and get the same sized implants, yet end up with completely different looking boobs.

Implants come in lots of sizes and shapes. The typical method for measuring implant size is by volume, usually measured in cubic centimeters or "CCs".

The surgeon's expertise is crucial when it comes to picking the implant size. He will probably give her some freedom of choice on the exact volume once he has suggested a general range.

There are several ways to help the surgeon suggest the right implants for your woman.

Finding Good Pictures

Keep looking for good pictures of great breasts that look like the ones your woman wants. "A picture is worth a thousand words", so showing a few photos to the surgeon will greatly help him to pick the right size.

Just what you need, an excuse to look at pictures of boobies on the internet!

Since the surgeon can't really tell much about the models in the pictures (height, weight, chest circumference, rib cage shape), you cannot rely on the pictures alone. They will, however, help him understand the "look" she wants.

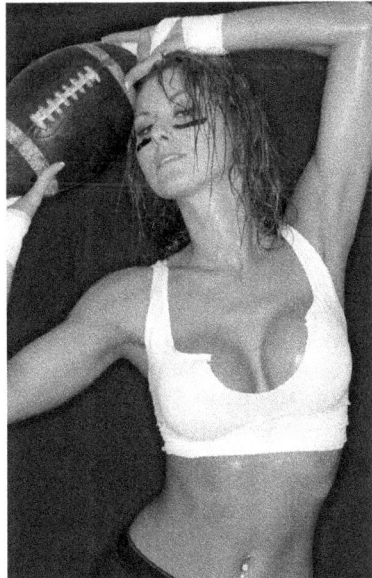

Practicing Your Plays

Here's a fun way to test out various implant volumes.

First, have her buy some cheap bras of various larger sizes. Have her put one one and put a sandwich baggie in between each breast and the big bra's cups. Fill each bag with dry rice until the cup is full. Then have her put on a shirt.

Now she should have some terribly fake-looking breasts in the next size up. Does she look totally unnatural? Does it look like she could go bigger? Talk to her about what each of you see and think. Take some photos.

Bra Band Size	Volume to Go Up One Cup
32"	100-200 CCs
34"	150-250 CCs
36"	200-300 CCs
38"	250-350 CCs

Repeat this with different sized bras until you find a size that is roughly what you both think is right. If she's a B-cup, try a C-cup bra, a D, and maybe even a DD. Find the size that she likes the best. It helps if you take a series of photos at each cup size to later compare them. She can later show the pictures of her desired outcome to her surgeon.

To get a very rough idea of the volume of implant she needs to reach her desired goal, measure the volume of rice in the bag. Pour the rice into a measuring cup. Use the conversion factor: 1 ounce is roughly 28 CCs. A cup is 8 ounces, or 237 CCs. With implants, one "bra cup" is approximately 175-200 CCs, but that depends on her chest size.[10]

Keep in mind that this bag-o-rice test is a VERY ROUGH indicator of the right size, so don't be worried if the rice bag looks bulgy. Some women prefer to use an old pair of pantyhose instead of a baggie.

---

10 Loftus. (p. 138)

If all that sounds like a real pain, there's now an easier way for your woman to gauge the approximate implant size she wants. One of the major implant makers, Allergan, has a line of implants known as Natrelle™, and now sells a "Natrelle™ Pre-Consultation Kit".

This kit includes a booklet and DVD providing your woman with the basics of breast augmentation and how to use the rest of the kit. The real value of the kit is that it comes with an adjustable "profile bra" and four implant sizers. These sizers are implant-shaped plastic bags filled with water and labeled 1-4.

All your woman needs to do is put the "profile bra" on over her bra, and insert two of the four implant sizers. She then can slip on various tops to see how the sizers make her look. She can then figure out which of these sizers is closest to giving her the look she wants. This might mean a fashion show that will make you drool!

Only one of each size implant is included in the kit. As your woman looks at herself in the mirror, she will be lopsided, but this might be helpful for comparing the different sizes.

The kit costs $40 plus shipping as of this printing. It can be found at *www.natrelle.com*.

Working with the Surgeon on Volume

Good communication between surgeon and patient is important for getting the right implants. It may require a lot of back-and-forth. Your woman and her surgeon may not choose the exact size implant until her pre-op appointment or the morning of the surgery.

Picking the exact volume is complicated, as it is based not only on your woman's breast size. Other decisions she makes about the implants (implant material, incision location, implant position) impact the size she can choose, and other factors, such as the circumference and shape of her chest can impact what will look best on her.

Implant Profile, Shape, and Surface

To be honest, this is pretty complicated. The surgeon is the best at helping her pick out which profile, shape, and texture of implant to choose. These choices are closely related to the implant volume.

Picking the right implant is an art, and the "right size" is very particular to each woman's body type, measurements, and desires.

Implant Profile

There are different "profiles" or "projections" of implants which dictate how much they stick out to the front. Some are relatively flat and some are middle of the road. Others stick out really far to give the girl a really curvy profile. Basically, the profile determines if her new look will make you say "wow", "WOW!", or "Va-va-va-VOOM!"

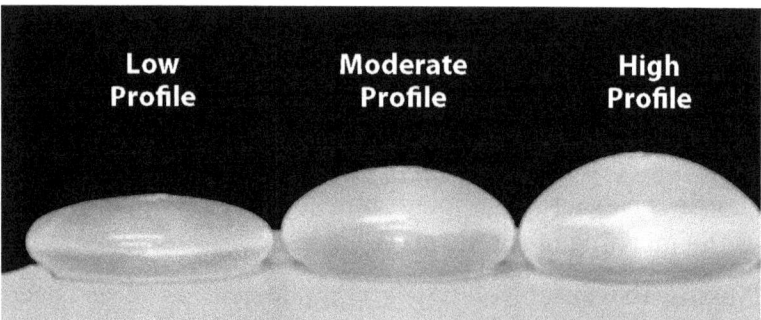

Allergan™ implant profiles
(Mentor™ calls their profiles by different names)

Implant Shape

There are two basic implant shapes, round or "teardrop"-shaped.

Round implants are simply round (a.k.a. "radially symmetric"). They look the same no matter which way they are rotated. Due to this shape, augmented breasts can look rather full above the nipple... but it also means they look the same even if the implant rotates within the pocket.

On the other hand, teardrop-shaped implants have more filler material in the lower part than in the upper part. This makes augmented breasts look more natural than round implants do. That is why they are also known as "anatomical" implants.

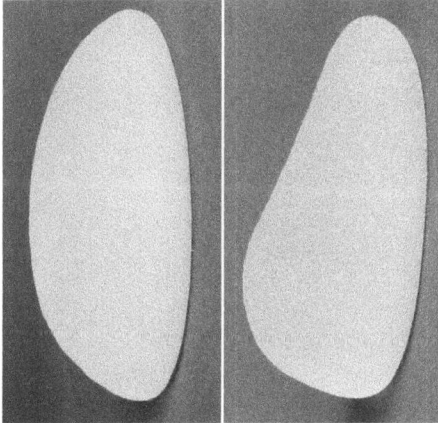

Implants can be either rounded or teardrop shaped

The downside to teardrop implants is that they may not remain in the proper orientation within her body. If they rotate, they can look strange, like her boob is sideways or upside-down. This is very rare, and usually only happens as a result of trauma or shock to breast. Unfortunately, once a rotation happens, revision surgery is needed to fix it. Anatomical implants can cost about $200 more than round implants.[11]

---

11 Loftus. (p. 134)

Implant Surface

The outer part of an implant can be smooth silicone poly-mer or it can have some texture. The texture helps teardrop implants stay oriented correctly in the body. Textured im-plants typically cost $100 more than smooth ones. [12]

No conclusive research has been done, but many doctors feel that smooth implants have a lower risk of seromas (a type of complication) and showing "traction" ripples. On the other hand, some doctors think that textured implants reduce the likelihood of capsular contracture (another type of complication).

The surgeon will likely have a suggestion for your lady re-garding the texture. She should discuss this with him.

---

12 Loftus. (p. 133)

* 12 *

The Play Call: Final Details

Booking the Surgery Date

Once she's chosen a surgeon and made her implant decisions, she will need to schedule the surgery. Doctors usually have to share operating rooms, so they can't just do surgery whenever they want. You'll probably have to book the surgery days, weeks, or maybe even months in advance.

She should pick a time that works for both of your schedules. If you can't get the time off the day of the surgery and a couple days afterward, you should get someone to take care of her. She should make sure has a close friend or relative available to help her through her first few days post-op if you can't or don't want to be there.

She should also make sure that she doesn't have any weddings or travel coming up within a few weeks of the surgery. She may be in pain for awhile, and will probably not want to be seen in a swimsuit immediately. But if push comes to shove, she CAN travel on a airplane. There is no risk of her implants "popping" because of the pressure change.

Also, if you have children, it's best if they stay with someone else while she has the surgery and recovers. They don't need to see mommy in her post-op state, and she won't be able to easily care for them.

Send them to sleep-away camp, a friend's house, or to their grandparents'.

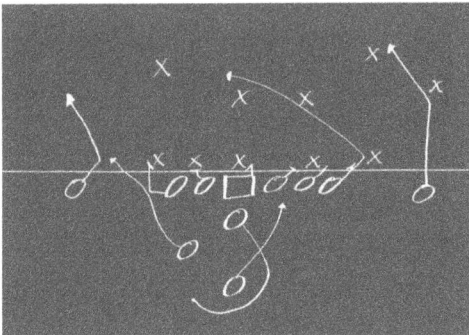

Otherwise, man, be ready to take care of the kids on your own and tell them, "Mommy is sick and needs to rest". Be prepared to do what you would if she had a really bad case of the flu.

A small price to pay for some new eye-candy!

Dr. Vip Says... Your prospective surgeons might discuss additional minor procedures that need to be done in addition to the augmentation. This doesn't mean they are trying to "up-sell" you. These minor procedures could include a crescent lift (if there is a sag to her breasts), areolar reduction, or nipple repair. Most surgeons do not charge additional fees for these procedures, as these procedures are also utilized to perform the breast augmentation.

Paying the Deposit

Most surgeons will require some money down to reserve the operating room and the surgical staff. That way your woman is discouraged from backing out at the last minute.

They may require anywhere from **$200-$500** to reserve the surgery time. They want this money up front when you are reserving the date.

The remaining cost of surgery is usually due at the pre-op appointment. Some doctors will require to be paid in full anywhere from two weeks before to the day of the surgery (especially if there is no pre-op appointment).

Dr. Vip Says... Once the consultation is completed, the two of you will agree on a surgical date and proceed with the preoperative work-up, which will include blood work and, in some cases, a pregnancy test, EKG, and chest x-ray. Some decisions about lab work to be performed depend on the woman's age and past medical and surgical history, while other labs are standard for that doctor. In most cases, your health insurance will cover this lab work, even though the rest of the procedure isn't covered.

Attending the Pre-Op Appointment

Once the surgery date is picked, the surgeon will likely schedule a pre-op appointment one or two weeks before the surgery. Then again, some surgeons don't do this.

In the pre-op appointment, the surgeon will likely:

- Review her desires and surgical choices
- Conduct a general medical exam (usually with blood tests)
- Give her the prescriptions for the painkillers
- Suggest any equipment to buy (such as special bras)
- Review all the important info she needs
- Have her fill out paperwork
- Collect payment for deposit on the surgery
- Answer any remaining questions

If she hasn't yet finalized the details of her boob job, the doc will help her make the choices at the pre-op appointment. If she's still up in the air about volume, he may have her try on a set of "sizers", which are special implants that she can

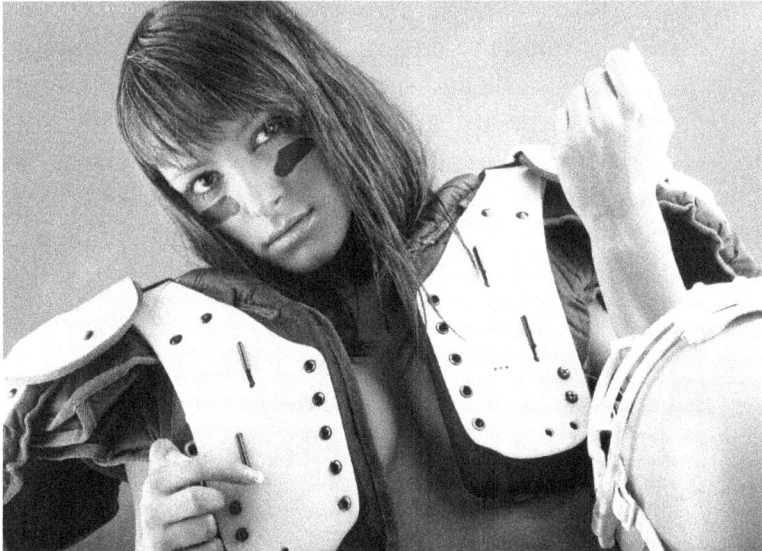

> Here are a few pointers about the pre-op appointment:
>
> Most surgeons write the necessary prescriptions the day of the consultation so your woman is ready with her medications on the day of the operation.
>
> The surgeon will review the labs and any other tests for abnormalities and the surgery will be scheduled definitively.
>
> The deposit to hold your surgery date varies between practices. Some doctors ask for 50% while others ask for $500 or $1,000. Most ask for $500 or more.
>
> Avoid taking aspirin or other NSAIDs (Advil, Motrin, Aleve), Vitamin E, or other herbal or vitamin supplements that can thin the blood.
>
> If your woman suspects that she has any tape, adhesive, latex, or iodine allergies, she should bring it up now so the nurses don't use it on her skin.
>
> Also, if your woman has any addiction history that worries you, be sure you discuss this with the surgeon when he gives you the pain medication prescriptions at the last pre-op visit, so that he can prescribe alternatives.
>
> The final pre-op visit is a great time to ask any lingering questions about follow-up appointments, exercising, physical activity, sexual activity and other limitations.

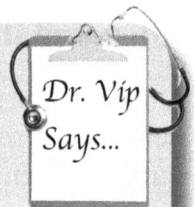

Dr. Vip Says...

wear in her bra to gain an understanding of how it would be to have different size breasts.

The medical exam is to ensure that she is healthy enough to undergo anesthesia and surgery. This can be very important, as it could be a deal-breaker. If he finds something to suggest she can't handle the surgery, then it's better to know now then to find out the hard way on the operating table. She should leave the pre-op appointment confident in what she's doing and excited to see the results.

Again, you can attend the pre-op if you want. The surgeon may ignore you again, and you may have to endure his looking at her boobs again. But if you're there to help support your woman, it can only strengthen your relationship.

Recording The Decisions

Once she's worked with her surgeon and made all the decisions, there's a very important step – recording the decisions and the rationale behind them.

Having a record of why she chose to get implants, why that particular surgeon, and why those exact implant details will be helpful. During her recovery, when she is under the influence of pain or medication (or just frustrated with a lengthy recovery), she may begin to regret the breast augmentation or the size she chose.

That's precisely when having a record is invaluable. You'll have something to remind her that it all made sense before she was suffering, and that it will be worth it in the end. It can also help to lift her spirits when she's low.

There are many ways of making this record. She can make a voice recording using a dictaphone, her cell phone's voicemail system, or computer software. Or she can record a short video explaining it all. She also could just write or type a

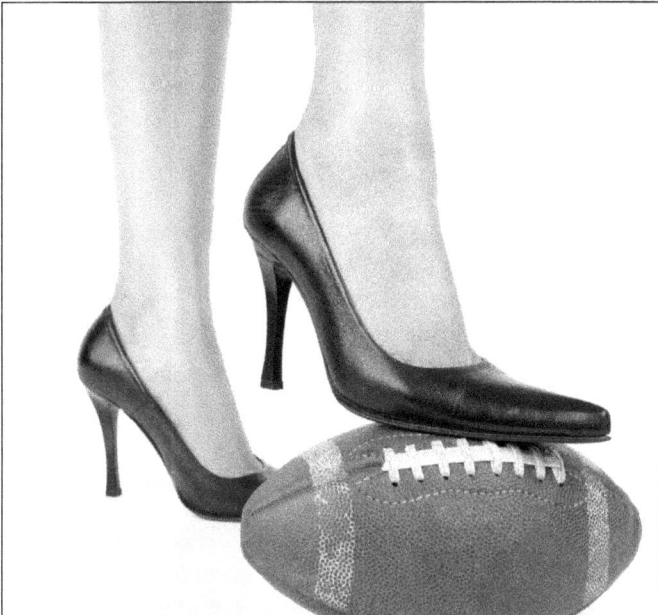

short note to herself.

If none of that seems to work for you, I've put together a "Reminders to Herself" worksheet that she can fill out. Download it at

www.FootballAndBoobs.com/reminders

Keep in mind that if your woman cancels, she may lose most or all of her deposit, depending upon how much notice she gives the surgeon. The doctor has to reserve the surgery suite, the time of the surgery technician, the RNs, and the anesthesiologist, who will need to be paid if it the surgery is cancelled last-minute.

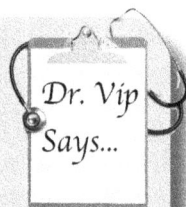

Dr. Vip Says...

If your woman is sick the week of her surgery, she should call the surgeon's office and to ask if the doctor wants her to come in. Some illnesses require that the procedure be postponed, while others will not. Do not wait until the last minute (the day prior to surgery) to call with concerns about a cold or other illness.

QTR

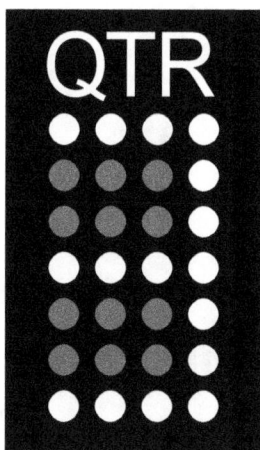

THIRD QUARTER: THE BIG PLAY

Questions this Section Answers:

What do we need to do to **prepare** for her surgery?

What do we need to do on **surgery day**?

What happens during the **first few days of recovery**?

How can I make her initial **recovery more pleasant** for us both?

What are the **signs of complications** that I should look out for?

How long will I have to wait to **see and play with her new boobs**?

13

The Cadence: Surgery Prep

Ok, let's review. Your woman is going to get a boob job. She knows who her surgeon will be, and most of the choices have been made.

Are you excited yet? Sure, the surgery may still be weeks away, but I bet the visions of her with a new set of sweater kittens are already dancing in your head!

In the days and weeks before Jane's surgery, I remember how I felt. I was like a kid in mid-December, everywhere I looked, there was something that reminded me of the "presents" that were about to come my way in my own special "Christmas".

Maybe you are like me, and all this boobie talk has you ready to look and play with your two newest friends. On the other hand, if your woman is talking non-stop about the surgery, you may be annoyed and just want it to be over with. Or you could just be nervous about what **might** happen during or after the surgery.

No matter how you feel, you should realize that it's okay for you to have some strong feelings about this big change. Yes, you are a man, but you have emotions too. Acknowledge them.

Ok, done yet? Now let's move on to the facts.

You want her new breasts to look the best they possibly can, don't you?

You want your woman to be as happy as possible before, during, and after the surgery, right?

You want her to heal as fast as possible so that you can look and play with the "new ladies" sooner, don't you?

Ok, good. To achieve those things, you will need to put in a little effort taking care of her before and after the surgery. You must also exercise patience. Her breasts will not be ready for playtime immediately after surgery, and will probably take weeks or maybe even months to look really good.

Don't worry. All that effort will pay off when you have a happier, more confident woman. When she feels sexier, dresses sexier, and maybe even has a higher libido, you will forget all about the time you spent taking care of her.

Do the right things to prepare and care for your woman. She will heal faster, her breasts will look better, you both will be happier, and your relationship will be stronger!

Football teams practice their plays hundreds of times only to run them a few times in the game. They watch hours of game film of each upcoming opponent so they can learn their tendencies, strengths, and weaknesses.

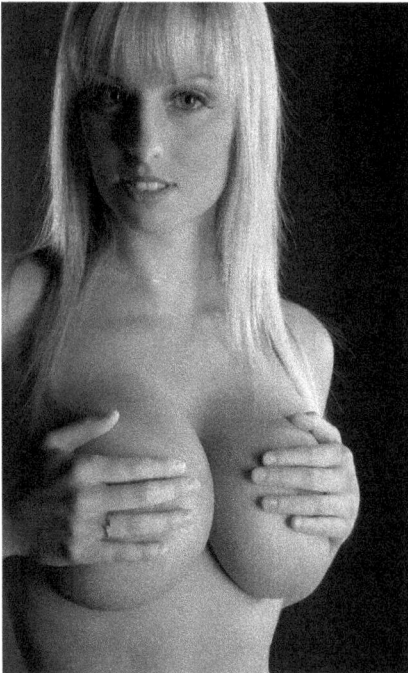

In other words, they prepare. Usually, surgeries are scheduled weeks or months in advance. Waiting for the surgery day will give you plenty of time to work out the details and prepare as needed. There is a lot you can both do before the surgery to make everything go more smoothly on surgery day, and the first few days after.

First, determine who will be her caretaker and make arrangements accordingly. Next, you need to set up your (or her) home, focusing especially on the area in which she will be staying while she recovers. Food needs to be prepared, and there are many supplies to be purchased that will be life savers. You'll also need to make sure that each of you is mentally ready and that she is physically ready.

"Down": Become Her Caretaker or Find One

Your woman needs a caretaker for her surgery. On operation day and for the next few days after, your woman will not be able to move around very well with new implants stuffed up into her chest. Simple things like opening doors, pulling back bed covers, buttoning her jeans, or even sitting up can be very difficult. And there's no way she can drive herself home after surgery.

Some men are very hands-on with their woman and want to be there to take care of them post-operatively. I highly recommend that you be your woman's caretaker if you have the time and patience.

Doing this will show her how much you care, and will score big points with her. She may not show it while she's recovering, but she will really appreciate your care and attention. Don't worry, she will show you just how much she appreciated it once she's better!

There is a lot you can both do before the surgery to make everything go more smoothly...

If for whatever reason, you can not be her caretaker, you should be ready and willing to help her find one. You will have to let your lady know that you can't or aren't willing to be there for her when she has her surgery. She may be relieved to have someone else help her.

She may ask you to find the caretaker, but more than likely

she will be more than happy to find a friend, family member, or hired help to take care of her.

If for some reason a friend or family member can not be her caretaker, or if she does not have anyone she wants to do it, you can hire a caregiver. There are nurses who specialize in post-cosmetic-surgery care.

A nurse is medically trained, knows the what to look out for and what to do should a complication arise. Hiring a nurse can make her recovery go more smoothly for you both. You won't have to be at your woman's beck and call, and you won't have to see her in pain. Win-win!

A good nurse will probably cost between $100 and $300 per day. If it really comes down to needing a nurse, you should get a reputable one. It will be worth it to have your woman well taken care of and to know that any and all complications will be dealt with properly.

Regardless of whether or not it will be you, someone will need to care for your woman immediately after surgery and for a couple of days after. Arranging for a caretaker may take some time due to personal schedules, so this should be your first step of preparation.

"Set": Preparing Your Home

Chances are that after surgery, your woman will need to rest for a few days up to a week. For the first day or two, she may be completely out of commission.

She will probably need to have food, medicine, and entertainment brought to her. Think of it like she's getting a bad case of the flu.

To make caring for her as easy as possible and to help her be as independent as possible, you two should to prepare your home for her recovery.

By "you two", I mean *she* will likely get really excited and start arranging things around the house as she is in her "nesting period" before the big day.

Your job is really simple. **Help her around the house when she asks for it.**

If she forgets something, it's okay to bring it up in a sensitive way, but don't tell her she's wrong because she hasn't done something listed here.

The major areas she will need to prepare are: 1) her recovery area, 2) the bathroom, and 3) the kitchen.

Preparing Her Recovery Area

After major surgery, her body will need to rest a lot. She will need a good place to sit and sleep at a 45 degree angle to keep the swelling down to a minimum.

Your woman's recovery area should have the following characteristics:

- Easy for her to sleep on her back with her chest elevated
- Convenient for staying entertained
- Small table nearby for food, water, and medicine
- Near a bathroom
- Near where you (or the caretaker) will be sleeping
- In a clean, non-depressing area

There are three main options for her sleeping area:

- Bed with MANY pillows
- Recliner
- Couch

Bed

Most women prefer sleeping in bed as they recover. If your woman chooses to do so, it will ensure that you are near her in case she needs you in the middle of the night. To keep her elevated at the required 45 degree angle on the bed, you can make a "pillow fort" to support her back, arms, and head.

Pillows are also useful for protecting her. If you move a lot when you sleep, putting several pillows between you may keep you from rolling over in the middle of the night and flopping an arm right onto her sensitive boobs.

Between the support and the protection, it's a good idea to have a stash of pillows on hand in case your woman needs more than expected.

Jane and I did some testing before her surgery and realized it would take all the pillows in the house to support her adequately on the bed, so we thought of an alternative.

The best thing that we found to keep her chest elevated was to get her a "husband" pillow. This is a little portable couch with soft arm-rests that look like arms that are hugging her.

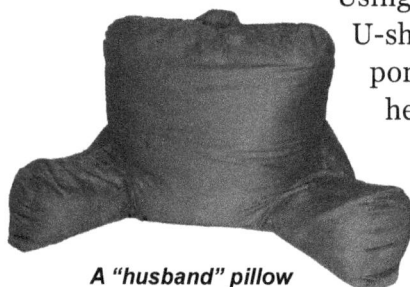

A "husband" pillow
Is convenient for her recovery

Using the husband pillow and a U-shaped neck pillow (to support her head against the head board), Jane was able to arrange a comfy supportive area on her bed that only took a few pillows. This left one pillow for me to sleep on, so I was happy about that.

The husband pillow is also really convenient for anytime you need to sit up on the bed or floor. If you buy one for the surgery, you might find it useful when playing on the floor with your kids, when playing video games, or reading Sports Illustrated while in bed.

Another option that may be more attractive to you is to buy *The Liberator.* This a fabric-covered wedge-shaped piece of foam that is sold as a "marital aid". It is made to be used for having sex in different positions, but I notice that it looks a lot like the wedges they use in athletic trainer's rooms to help people recline while receiving treatment. I think that investing in one of these "to help with her recovery" (wink, wink) could be worth the price. Then later on, you can use it for some wild times!

Recliner or Couch

As great as recliners are for watching football, they are even better for breast augmentation recovery. They can let her sit up or lean back for sleeping. Since they are usually pointed at a TV, this can help to keep her entertained so you can maybe go to work or grab a beer with your buddies while she rests.

If a recliner isn't an option, the couch is another good spot for her recovery area. Like a recliner, most couches tend to be near a TV, so your woman should be able to stay entertained while recovering.

However, couches can be pretty rigid and narrow, and usually aren't the most comfortable place to sleep for extended periods.

Whether she chooses the bed, the recliner, or the couch, the bottom line is that she needs to be supported.

Now that you have the basics of reclining relaxation arranged, you need to work on the rest.

Table

Wherever she'll be recovering, there are a bunch of things that she will need have within easy reach. Make sure there's some kind of small *table* at arm level nearby. A night stand, end table, or TV tray are great choices.

First, a bottle or glass of *water* should always be on the table. Also, keep a small *snack* of easily digestible food near her.

Think of the food she feeds you when you have the flu. Very plain stuff like crackers works well.

Keep her **pills** on the table too, preferably without the child-proof caps. She needs her pecs to open them, so they can be very difficult for her to open post-op.

She will need to take certain pills at certain times, so I've created a handy medicine log that you can download from

www.FootballAndBoobs.com/medicine

I recommend that you print this log out and keep it on the table next to the medicine.

To make it easier for her to communicate with the outside world, she will probably want to put a house phone or cell **phone** on the table too.

Last but not least, keep her entertained. Think *Sex and the City* or *The Notebook* on **DVD/BluRay**, a pile of trashy romance novels, or celebrity gossip **magazines**. Whatever she's into, make sure it is on hand so she can focus on something other than the pain she might be in. If she forgot or didn't have time to do this, and you remember to pick up stuff that she really cares about, you will score big points.

Whatever she's into, make sure it is on hand so she can focus on something other than the pain she might be in.

A **laptop** is a good idea too. It can keep her entertained and connected to the outside world.

If she wears **glasses**, you should keep them nearby, as she probably won't want to put in her contact lenses.

Two more quick things that men have noted as important for her recovery area. A **nightlight** will make it easier for you to dispense her pills and to walk her to the bathroom when she needs to go right after you just fell asleep.

For the first day or two she may be nauseated, so you may

need a puke bucket near the bed. A small trash can with a bag, a paper bag, a bucket, or a coffee can (with lid) all make great vomit receptacles.

Preparing the Bathroom

Compared to the recovery area, preparing the bathroom will be simple, but it's still important.

Again, your woman will probably be taking care of all this, but if she forgets or does not have time, you might need to help her.

She won't be able to reach up high, so keep things she needs down on the counter. The most important things to keep there are:

- Toilet Paper
- Towels
- Toothbrush and Toothpaste
- Deodorant
- Any makeup she "can't live without"
- Feminine hygiene products (as needed)

During her recovery, if she goes to pee and ends up with her butt in the water, she will be angry with you. Also, lifting the lid may be difficult for her. For the time being, **THE TOILET SEAT STAYS DOWN and the TOILET LID STAYS UP!!**

Preparing the Kitchen

The kitchen is another area that will need preparation. After the surgery, she won't be able to reach up to high cabinets. She should put a plate, a glass, and whatever food she might want down on the counter for once she's up and about. The last thing you want is for her to try to reach up and injure herself or harm the outcome of her surgery.

Food

Your woman should make it easy for her caretaker to feed her.

She should buy foods that are easy to digest for the first day, like jello, crackers, meal-replacement shakes, and soup.

After her stomach is settled, she may be able to handle more normal food. Many women will choose to cook several meals ahead of time and freeze them so that they can easily be heated later.

If she didn't do this, you may have to cook for her or get some good take-out. If you must cook, you should buy food that YOU KNOW HOW TO COOK. Don't try to get fancy. If all you can do is sandwiches and oatmeal, then buy that. Clearly, you will be responsible for feeding the kids if they are at home.

Beverages

Keeping her well-hydrated will be just as or more important than feeding her.

Her body is healing from major surgery, and she will need to drink a LOT of water. She needs to drink more than she thinks she should drink.

Make sure that she has some water available to drink at all times. You can also give her Gatorade or Pedialyte that to replace her electrolytes. Keep her away from soda for the first couple of days. Also, keep the booze away from her for a few weeks (based on surgeon's orders).

Also, while she is reclining, a **bendy-straw** will make drinking a lot easier for her.

Other Shopping

Your woman may need a lot of ice to help her heal faster and make the swelling go down so you can touch her boobs sooner!

Since she will probably need ice faster than most ice-makers can make it, it is wise to buy **re-freezable gel ice packs** (usually about 4"x6"). She will need these often, so just one won't work. You'll need many of them, probably 4. This way she can have one on each boob, and two others in the freezer ready to replace them.

Another great option is **frozen peas**. They mold to her body better than gel ice packs and are cheaper!

Right after surgery, there's only a slim chance your woman will be willing to wait in the car for you to get her pain medications from the pharmacy. It only makes sense to get the prescriptions filled as soon as the doc gives them to her. There also may be some medicines that the surgeon wants her to take before the surgery, so go to the pharmacy ASAP.

There are a few other things that one of you may want to pick up, depending on what the surgeon suggests. She should ask her surgeon about each of these.

Some surgeons recommend an herbal medication called "arnica montana" to help minimize bruising. These pills are usually taken 3 days before surgery and up to two weeks after surgery.

"Arnica gel" is a topical solution that is applied to bruises after surgery to help make them go away faster. It must be kept away from the incision site.

"Bromelain" is a natural enzyme (found in pineapple) that prevents and reduces swelling. It is found in fresh pineapple and any form of ginger. Usually, if a surgeon recommends it, he will advise her to take it in pill form.

She might also need one or more special bras for her recovery. Let her work with the surgeon on that. Most women agree that cotton is the most comfortable, and most surgeons are emphatic that they should not have an underwire. Some surgeons, like Jane's, suggest zip-in-front sports bras.

"Blue 42": Preparing Yourselves and Others

Once the caretaker and home are prepared, you must make sure your "team" is ready to go, both mentally and physically.

Mentally Preparing Yourself

If she hasn't already, your woman may soon start talking about *nothing but* breast implants. You may get to a point you never thought possible – tired of hearing about boobs. This is just a fact of life when dealing with a woman getting implants.

Your woman knows that she is undergoing a major change, and you need to be mentally ready too.

Most men in your position are excited about the upcoming surgery and new boobs. Many do not fully realize the effort and patience that will be required of them.

Let's be honest, it's really easy for us to get carried away and just think, "Boobies! Boobies! Great big boobies!"

Something like that kept running through my head in the days before Jane's surgery. I kept imagining what she would look like with our new "friends". I thought about looking at them and about playing with them. I thought about how happy she would be once she got them.

Some men are not so excited, especially if they don't agree with their woman's decision to get implants. It's a perfectly natural reaction to feel a little nervous (or a lot) about the situation.

Sometimes a man fears what might happen if something went wrong and his lady weren't around anymore. Such

> *It's a perfectly natural reaction to feel a little nervous (or a lot) about the situation.*

a man is afraid of the surgery changing his life drastically.

Questions race through his head, like:

- "What if she doesn't wake up?"
- "How will I care for the kids? "
- "What if the doctor really messes up her breasts?"
- "What if she starts wearing nothing but really sexy clothes and men start staring?"
- "What if she changes her mind and wants to leave me?"

The more the fearful man thinks about these questions, the more nervous he becomes, and the more irrational fear he will experience.

A smart person once explained that FEAR is nothing more than False Expectations Appearing Real. In other words, if you are thinking such thoughts, your brain may be a runaway train focusing on a highly unlikely situation.

If you are getting worried, do yourself a big favor. Stop. Take a deep breath. You can flip over to the section on "Complications" to see how unlikely each one is. This may reassure you.

If your worries are more about how your relationship might change, talk to her. She knows you and should be able to help you. Then again, you might not want to show her your fear if she is afraid too. This is up to you.

Hopefully, thinking about how slight the chances of a bad outcome are will calm you down. If not, I hope that talking with me, a friend, or a family member will ease your nerves. By doing it, you may find your fear transforming into excitement.

When Jane's surgery approached, I was more excited than I was nervous. I was not at all thinking about how much I would have to do to take care of her and how long it would take.

Thankfully, she had done all her homework and told me all about what the recovery would be like. I *knew* what to expect, but sometimes emotions are stronger than rational thought... even for men.

On surgery day, you will probably be nervous. Be ready for that. On the other hand, you must realize that you need to be strong to help keep her calm. Be the man; be supportive.

The first 24 hours after surgery may not be very pretty, and she may depend on you heavily for a few days. Be ready.

To be honest, when we got home from surgery, I realized that I was not fully mentally prepared to see her in such a state of pain and helplessness.

This was a big revelation for me, and really sparked me to write this book for you. You discover more about that in the "Initial Recovery" section. Be sure to read that section thoroughly so that you can start to comprehend what the recovery will be like. You won't really understand it until you're right in the middle of your woman's recovery, but that section will give you a taste.

If you want, I am willing to give you a free 15-minute consultation to help calm you down. Email me at

Dallas@FootballAndBoobs.com

to let me know your concerns and we can arrange a phone consultation.

Remember, there is work ahead of you. Accept that fact, and you will be golden. Be ready to see her in varying degrees of discomfort and helplessness, and be ready to hear many complaints.

Taking care of her will score you major points, and will increase the chance that you get to touch her boobies as much as you want!

Again, a few reminders:

- You may have to wait days to see or touch her boobs.
- You may have to wait weeks for sex.
- It may take months for her boobs to be fully ready.

ACCEPT THESE FACTS, and you will both benefit.

Ultimately, your attitude and reactions to her will be very important in helping her feel better and recover faster. While you are waiting to enjoy the fruits of your labor, you'll need to try your best to remain positive rather than show your frustration.

You can do it. You will earn those new boobies!

Helping Her Mentally Prepare

Just like you, your woman will probably be excited, nervous, or a combination of the two in the weeks and days leading up to her boob job. Talk to her about how she feels, and reassure her that she has made the right decision for herself.

If she gets really scared, you should do your best to comfort her. Talk

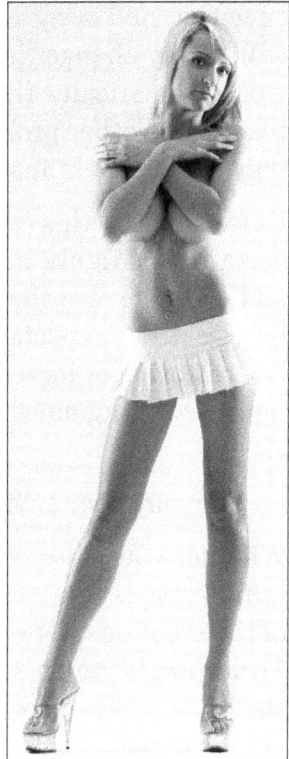

Not Overnight!

Her new breasts will NOT be perfect overnight, nor in a few days or weeks.

It may take **UP TO A YEAR** to see the final results.

Remember, this is a long, slow-developing touchdown play.

You must have patience. Accept that fact.

with her, and possibly suggest she re-read her "Reminders to Herself" worksheet from

www.FootballAndBoobs.com/reminders

Not all women get scared. Many are calm yet eager. Some get so excited that they lose touch with reality. These women get carried away and start to think that breast implants will totally change their lives. They think that the surgery will automatically fix deep-rooted self-esteem issues, or that all the other problems in their life will disappear once they change their appearance.

Unfortunately, this isn't the case. Breast implants may give her a better figure and more confidence, but they cannot and will not solve all of her issues. It is important for her to have realistic expectations and take this surgery for what it is – restoring or increasing her femininity by enhancing her figure. Nothing more.

If your woman is one of these "solve all my problems" women, you may need to help her face reality.

Whether you are easing her fears, talking her down from unrealistic expectations, or just helping her deal with any of the emotions between these extremes, one fact remains. **You should be talking with your woman** as much as she wants throughout the process. Discussing feelings is not most men's favorite topic, but it is important, and it will likely help her to feel better about her surgery.

Especially *focus on listening* to what she has to say. Not only does it help you understand her, but—more importantly—it makes her feel understood.

Women tend to be much more talkative than men, so too much conversation about feelings can be a little tiring for some of us. Tough it out. It's just another part of the small price you must pay for new boobs to play with!

Preparing Her Body

Since your woman is getting implants, she obviously cares about how her body looks. Hopefully, she also exercises regularly.

The more in shape she is in the days and weeks leading up to her surgery, the faster she will be able to recover.

One area she should focus on is her abs. The stronger her abs are, the easier it will be for her to sit up from a reclining position. Jane knows several friends who had great difficulty getting up on their own after surgery because they didn't have good abdominal strength. Some even ended up hurting their backs.

On the other hand, if your woman is getting "unders", she will want to **stop** doing any chest-strengthening exercises at least one month before surgery. The looser her pecs are, the easier it will be for them to stretch around the implant.

One big thing that can be hard to deal with is getting her off nicotine and booze. Many sur-

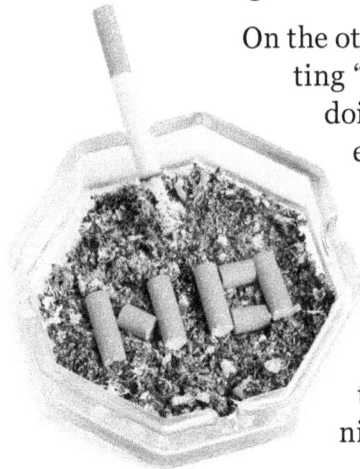

geons suggest that women stop smoking and drinking at least two weeks before the surgery and not start back up for at least two weeks after surgery. This will prevent complications and help her heal faster. Smoking reduces the oxygen in her blood and slows the healing process. Nicotine gum is no better, as it too inhibits healing. Alcohol inhibits her body's ability to absorb nutrition and this her blood, harming her recovery in two ways.

Also, there are some medications that your surgeon may ask her to not take in the days or weeks prior to surgery.

Finally, if your woman is over 35, her surgeon may require that she have a mammogram before her surgery.

Telling Other People

In my humble opinion, it's not really anyone's business whether or not your woman gets implants. However, there are some people who WILL notice her more ample figure and may ask questions.

If you have children, telling them can be difficult. Actually, YOU shouldn't have to tell your kids. Your woman should do it.

If the kids are very young (usually under <3 years old), they probably won't notice mommy's new knockers and don't need to be told. They probably won't remember even if they do notice.

For young children (3-8 or so), she might want to sit them down and tell them that mommy is doing something that will help her feel better. She may "have a boo boo" or may have "hurt her back" and won't be able to hug them tight or pick them up for a little while.

For older children who will notice mom's new knockers, the talk can be more delicate, especially if you have a teenage daughter.

Many young women have body-image issues and seeing their mother get implants may make your daughter question her body even more. There are many internet resources to help you and your woman know what to say. This conversation needs to be handled delicately and with love.

Tell the rest your family if you think it is appropriate. Do it if you need their support and don't think that they will be judgmental.

If she's careful about what she wears around her family, she might not need to say anything if she doesn't want to.

Ultimately, it's your family. I can not tell you what you or your woman should say or do. Just use your best judgment, and you will work it out.

Most women don't want the whole world to know about their implants and choose to keep the surgery secret. The two of you can tell anyone anything you want about her surgery. The big issue is making your stories match up. What do you say to the preacher, the little-league coach, your woman's mother, her boss, her friends, or her co-workers? It can get confusing if some people have the inside scoop and others don't. You don't need to tell anyone right now, but if you do, make sure you both keep your stories straight.

"White 19": The Night Before Surgery

There are three major things she need to do before surgery:
- Make sure her body is ready
- Make sure both of your minds are ready
- Perform last-minute preparations

To make it easy to remember this all, check out
www.FootballAndBoobs.com/night-before
The checklist there will help you.

Her Body's Intake

Whether it's rotator cuff repair for a quarterback or an ACL replacement for a running back, surgeons almost always require that the patient NOT eat or drink anything after midnight the night before surgery. This reduces the risks while under anesthesia.

No glass of water in the morning, no breakfast. Nothing in her system at all. You may have to be the "bad cop" that keeps her stomach empty. Be nice; don't eat in front of her if she is hungry.

Also, make sure she's had no alcohol, cigarettes, or forbidden medications, especially in the 48 hours leading up to the surgery.

Relaxation

The best mental state for her prior to surgery is one of relaxation. You can book her a massage the day before surgery or run her a nice bubble bath the night before. Either should help her to relax.

Another way to help you both relax is to have sex. Doing so releases chemicals in the brain that minimize anxiety, and the exercise is good for you both. Plus, you may not be having sex for two or more weeks after this, so get as much as you can now! Make sure that she showers afterward so that she goes into surgery squeaky clean.

Some men are nervous the night before their woman's surgery and can have trouble sleeping, due to a combination of fear, anxiety, and excitement. It's natural to be a little nervous. Do your best to get some rest though, because you will need to be on top of your game surgery day.

Last-Minute Prep

There are many last-minute preparations that are key to a successful boob job day. When you wake up, both of your nerves might be running high, so it's a good idea to set everything out the night before. That way you don't forget anything

First, make sure you have all the **paperwork and payment** ready to go. Most surgeons require these weeks before the surgery, but some wait until the day of surgery. If she has filled out the "Reminders to Herself" worksheet, bring it, too.

If you are driving her to and from surgery, you will want to get your car ready. Put a **pillow** in the car, with the paperwork and payment. Also, make sure you have a small bottle of **water** and some **facial tissue**.

Perhaps most importantly, put some sort of **puke-bucket** in the car. Use a trash can, bucket, grocery bag, or a coffee can with lid.

You may want to throw one of **her favorite CDs** in the car to help her relax and stay distracted before and after the surgery.

Also, you should bring a magazine, book, or laptop to keep you entertained while she is in surgery.

She might want you to take pictures of her boobs before the surgery. These will be valuable later, as she will be ale to compare her before and after shots to see how much she has really changed. Standard angles include head-on, profile, and diagonal (her 2 o'clock and 10 o'clock).

Finish preparing the house fully. You may have read the section about getting the kitchen, bathroom, and recovery area ready, but decided to leave your space as it was to keep living your life before surgery. Go ahead and put everything where it needs to be.

Make sure the ice packs or frozen peas are in the freezer. Remember to lay the ice packs flat.

She should make a **to-do list** of all the chores around the house that will need to be done.

Make sure all her **clothes for recovery** are easy to access, including her support bras, sweat pants, button-down shirts, and zip-up hoodies. Putting them in one drawer where you can easily grab them is wise.

Have her set out her surgery-day clothing at this point. She should have some loose pants, comfy, non-lace-up shoes, and a button-up or zip-up shirt or jacket.

Don't forget to set the alarm clock!

You should be all ready to go, now get to sleep. The play is about to start!

Remember, your lady can have nothing by mouth after midnight the night before surgery and take a couple of minutes to read through the pre-op packet that the surgeon's office gave her at the final visit before surgery.

On the day of the procedure, remember to arrive early so that the nurses can prepare her adequately and efficiently.

Dr. Vip Says...

* 14 *

The Play Begins: Surgery Day

Friend, you must realize one thing. This surgery is very important to your woman. She wants the results so badly that she is willing to make all of the physical, emotional, interpersonal, and financial sacrifices that are required.

On surgery day, she will begin a transformation—not only a physical transformation, but a mental and emotional one, too.

This transformation will not be immediate and will begin painfully.

Change is hard to deal with for most people. Remember the last time she bought the other kind of toothpaste? Undergoing a major change while being in physical pain is going to be even more difficult for your woman.

Some women can get bent out of shape under this burden. During the initial recovery period, your woman may behave differently than usual. She may be on an emotional roller coaster that could will affect her moods and behavior.

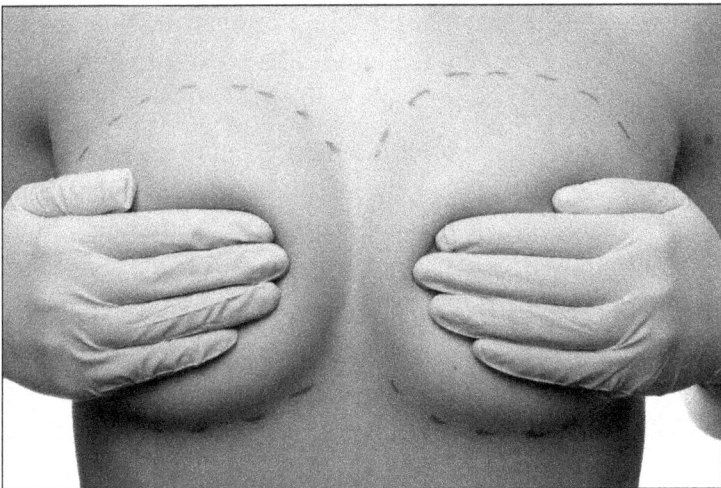

Some women worry incessantly, and convince themselves that something is horribly wrong when it isn't. Others turn into real witches, complaining about everything.

That's why you need to be the rock of your relationship. You must be calm, cool, and collected. You need to be the rational one. That's why you have this book, and this chapter in particular. It will guide you through the beginning of her recovery.

On the other hand, some women are even-keeled and behave the same in any situation. Hopefully, your woman will be like this and will even be happy with her not-yet-ready results. Just don't assume so, and be prepared to deal with her emotions.

Regardless of how the game is going, now is the time for the big play! Play it right and you two will win the game. Let's hope it all works out for you.

The play starts on the day of surgery, with your alarm clock going off.

"Hut, Hut, Hike!": Morning of Surgery

On this special morning, your woman will likely be abuzz with activity. She may be so excited or nervous that she forgets everything she has read and falls right into her normal morning routine.

While she's getting ready for surgery, make sure she DOES NOT PUT ON any make-up, perfume, hair products, moisturizer, deodorant, jewelry, high heels, tight shoes, boots, or contact lenses. She may complain, and feel very unsexy, but this is necessary for surgery.

Be sure to keep the food, drink, and cigarettes out of her body. No vitamins, no supplements, no water. Nothing enters her mouth. Make sure you've gotten all of the last-minute items taken care of.

If you're nervous, take a deep breath and get ready for a long day!

The Snap: Getting to the Surgical Facility

Once you've gotten everything loaded into the car, it's time to go!

On the way to the surgical facility, she will most likely be nervous because he has a lot of thoughts racing through her head. Depending on what your woman is like, she might be frozen in silence or running her mouth like Terrell Owens.

She might get cold feet and want to cancel. You might suggest she re-read the "Reminders to Herself" worksheet that she filled out to remember why she wants *this* surgery with *this* surgeon.

Whether she's a ball of nerves or just super excited, she'll need to be calm for the surgery. Hold her hand, or play a CD she likes. You know your woman better than anyone and will need to do what you think is best to keep her calm.

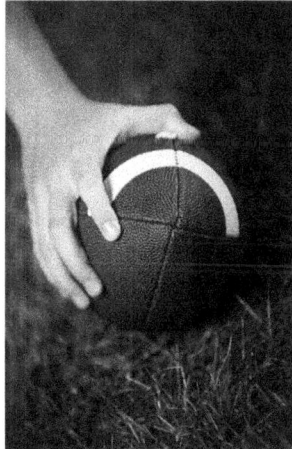

Even though you're acting calm, you may be really nervous. Some men have compared this to driving their wives to the hospital for childbirth. Only in this case, walking into the medical facility is a bit less rushed.

The Dropback: Waiting Together

You may have to sit in the waiting room of the surgical facility once you arrive or they may usher her directly into surgical prep.

If you have time to kill, there might be some before and after photos or magazines in the waiting room. If she looks like she needs something to take her mind off the moment, give her one to read.

Otherwise, hold her hand, hug her, and keep her calm. Do what's best for your woman.

Some men get so nervous that their women must comfort them! Hopefully, this won't be you!

While you are waiting, a nurse may give your woman a sedative to relax her before surgery. This will probably be right before...

The Throw: She Goes Into Surgery

Here it is. She just got called in for surgery, and is walking through the door. She may look back at you or she may just plow straight ahead. You will be left in the waiting room, nervous, and wondering what to do.

* 15 *

The Ball's Flight: During Surgery

On any deep pass, once the ball leave's the quarterback's hand, it is out of his control. There's nothing he can do to make it more successful, and there's not much the center can do either. It's all up to the receiver to get to the ball, catch it, and run it past the defense.

Similarly, once she's in the operating room, it's all out of your control and hers. It's all up to the surgeon and his staff.

Just like a deep pass spiraling through the air, the time while she is in surgery can be highly dramatic.

Waiting can be very nerve-wracking, but it doesn't have to be.

So that you don't go out of your mind with nervousness, you'll need to keep yourself entertained for 1-3 hours. Grab that book, magazine, mp3 player, or laptop that you put in the car, or you can go hang out somewhere until she's out of surgery.

Whether you are still in the waiting room or up the street at a coffee shop, they will call you once she is out of surgery.

Your woman will have an IV inserted so that the anesthesiologist can sedate her prior to bringing her into the operating room. Prior to sedation, the anesthesiologist will speak to both of you and tell you what to expect before, during, and after the surgical procedure.

Dr. Vip Says...

Prior to sedation, the surgeon will "mark" the patient—this is the surgeon's road map. He will also mark where the incisions will be. Your girl will then be sedated and taken into the operating room. The surgery can take anywhere from 45 minutes to 1.5 hours. Some surgeons prefer to wrap patients afterwards, some place surgical bras, or some prefer nothing but simple gauze. Once the procedure has been completed, she will remain in the recovery for a few hours before she is released home.

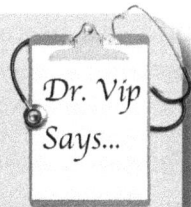

They will let you know how she is doing and whether or not you can see her immediately.

You might have to wait even longer. After the surgery, they will probably keep her in a recovery room for 1-2 hours, depending on how she is doing.

They will then call you again when she is all ready to go home. When you first see her, she will probably be in pain and look like she's still half asleep.

This will not be a sexy moment. As excited as you may be, do not expect to see her boobs anytime soon. They will most likely be wrapped up or hidden in a bra for a few days.

Be sympathetic... Just tell her that you love her and everything will be better soon.

Be sympathetic. Don't say something stupid like, "I bet that hurts" or, "You look like crap". Just tell her that you love her and everything will be better soon. Try to help her and take care of her.

Make sure that you get the "implant package insert". It may be in her hands, or you may have to ask the staff for it. This card will list the brand, size, lot number, and serial numbers of the implants that were put in her body. This info will be really important to have if she ever needs a revision surgery down the line, so make sure to keep it in a safe place.

The next task is getting her into your car for the ride home.

When I picked Jane up from the recovery room after surgery, she was in pain. She was half asleep and wrapped up like a mummy.

The nurse pushed her in a wheelchair as I walked next to her. We took the elevator down to my car, which I had pulled up to the loading zone.

I remember how difficult it was for her to climb into the

passenger's seat of my car. This was a sad sight, and it hurt me to see her like that. She was not happy at all. Hopefully your lady will have an easier time.

Once your woman is in the seat, position the pillow however she is most comfortable, buckle her in, and put the puke bucket on the floor or in her lap so it remains accessible and is strategically positioned.

On the drive home I tried going as slowly and smoothly as possible, but every time I turned at all or hit a tiny bump, Jane squealed in pain a little.

Your woman may not be in as much pain on the ride home, but she will still probably notice every bump in the road. Do your best to make it smooth sailing, or be ready to hear moans and whimpers. If not, tell her how tough she is!

Don't plan on making any stops on the way home, unless she really wants to and feels good.

Once you get home, help her out of the car and to her recovery area. Get her some water, and a light snack if she needs to take some pills. Start using the "Medicine Log" as soon as she takes her first meds, and keep it up according to surgeon's orders.)

Chances are that she will want to do nothing but sleep for the first couple of hours.

If she is nauseated, keep the puke container close to her. The greatest risk for her to be sick is the first few hours after returning home. If she does feel ill, remind her that it will pass.

Hopefully, she will have fallen asleep by now and you can take a few minutes to relax.

This is the beginning of her intense recovery period, when she needs you the most. Now is the time for you to really earn your right to those boobs!

Dr. Vip Says...

It is common for each woman to react slightly differently to anesthesia. Although Dallas is wise to remind you to bring that puke pot, most surgeons do give their patients medication both before and during the procedure to limit postoperative nausea and vomiting. Just in case, you might think about driving to and from surgery in *her* car...

* 16 *

The Catch: Initial Recovery

O nce she's out of surgery, there will be three major phases to her recovery.

The first 1-3 days will be intense recovery, and require you (or her caregiver) to wait on her hand and foot. Then, up to the first week post-op she may still need help and lots of rest, but she will be less dependent on you. After that, during the weeks and months post-op, she will be back to 100%, but will still need patience to wait for her boobs to fully heal.

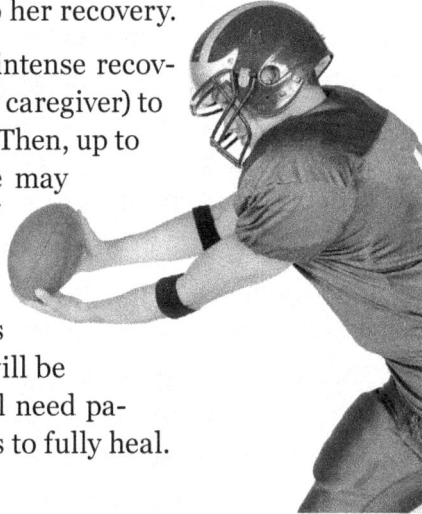

Tucking the Ball: The First Few Days

Expect her to stay in bed, on the couch, or in the recliner the rest of surgery day, and maybe even the next few days. During this time, she may need your help for everything: taking her medication, walking to the bathroom, showering, changing clothes, possibly even feeding herself.

Then again, some women have very easy recoveries. So your woman may be up on a shopping spree the very next day. I just want to make sure that you are well-prepared no matter what.

How long she is down for the count depends on a combination of her sur-

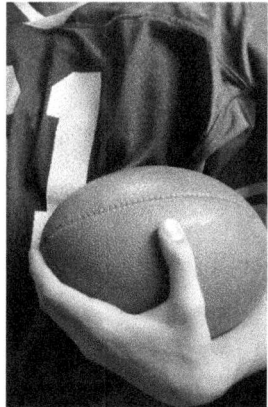

geon's skill, the procedure she chose, her pain threshold, her health, and her reaction to the surgery and any medication she takes.

After the first days of feeling like she was hit by a truck, she will likely probably start feeling better and be able to do more activities her own. She will be happy to start sitting up on her own, but she may still need help with things like putting away dishes and washing her hair.

There are several things you will likely notice about her. These are several of the most common issues you will encounter: what you'll see, what she'll feel, and what you can do to help her.

Pain

After her anesthesia wears off, she will likely be in pain. She may wince, make noises, or complain.

The best thing you can do to help her pain is to stay on top of her medication schedule.

Her boobs hurt as her body does three things:
- Overcomes the trauma of the pocket creation
- Adjusts to the implant stretching her tissues and muscles
- Heals the incisions

Her back may also be hurting her from hours or days of reclining and from not being able to stand fully upright due

Once you get your lady home, you will have medications to give her. The most common medications are Vicodin, Darvocet, Percocet, and Tylenol with codeine for pain; Flexeril or Robaxin for muscle tension; and Keflex, Cipro, or another antibiotic for protection against infection. It is important to take these for pain, and it is very important to take the full course of antibiotics that are prescribed.

Dr. Vip Says...

Take note that some women will feel nauseated from the pain medications. If this happens, call the surgeon and ask for prescription-strength Tylenol.

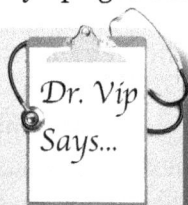

to pectoral tightness. She'll be surprised by how much she needs her pecs everyday!

Her boobs and back will most likely hurt the most when she wakes up in the morning.

Surgeons prescribe pain medication to help women as they recover from breast augmentation. While these can be powerful drugs, do not worry. Typically a surgeon will only give a woman enough pain pills for the first week, so there isn't much risk of her getting addicted to them.

That being said, if your woman wants to be clear-headed sooner, she should wean herself off the pain pills and start using Tylenol (acetaminophen). She SHOULD NOT take aspirin or ibuprofen (like Advil), as these can thin her blood and cause complications.

Some surgeons will also send women home with a "pain pump". No, this is not the shoe Sarah Sherman used to kick you in the junk at that 8th grade dance. This is a pump attached to a tube that runs into her incision to administer the pain medication directly to the wound. If your woman gets the pain pump, she will need to return to the surgeon a few days later for removal.

Remember, it is your responsibility to wake her up every few hours to take her pain pills and any antibiotics the surgeon has prescribed.

Remember, it is your responsibility to wake her up every few hours to take her pain pills and any antibiotics the surgeon has prescribed. Stay on top of the pain; don't wait until the pain is bad before giving her the pain pills. They do take a little while to kick in. Make sure she takes ALL the antibiotic pills she's been prescribed, which is important to fighting off infections. In fact, not finishing all of the antibiotics can even cause her to get a worse infection later.

To keep you from forgetting when she needs medicine, it makes sense to set an alarm clock or a countdown timer (like on your microwave or cell phone). Whenever it goes off, you should wake her and give her the pills, a snack, and water.

Sometimes she will be in more pain than at other times, so she may need the pain pills before the alarm says she should. Give the medicine to her whenever she asks, but not more often than once every 2-3 hours (or whatever the bottle says).

Frozen peas or ice packs can also help with the pain by reducing the swelling. They should never be placed directly on her skin as it can cause ice burns, so she should have a towel or extra T-shirt between the cold packs and her skin. Icing is most effective for the first 72 hours post-op.

To help her back pain, you can put a heating pad or hot water bottle under her back for up to an hour at a time. This will help loosen her back muscles. It is important that you do not get the heat anywhere near her boobs, as heat increases swelling.

Talk to her about her pain if she wants. Be sympathetic and remind her that it's normal to be in pain. It's expected.

On the other hand, try to entertain her so she keeps her mind on something other than the pain. Give her the remote control, and let her watch all the E! and Lifetime she wants. Put her favorite DVD in the player, give her a book to read, or put a pile of magazines right next to her. It's much better for her movies to annoy you than it is for her be bored and in pain.

Swollen and High

The first few days and weeks after the surgery, your woman's breasts probably will be like Cheech Marin and Tommy Chong with a half pound of Maui Wowee: very high.

They may look like they are in a mega-push-up bra. They may look very "square-ish" and up around her chin. Jane's breasts looked like this immediately after her surgery and stayed this way for a few weeks. Your job is to NOT say anything bad about them.

In addition to being high up on her chest, her boobs may look stretched tight and shiny due to swelling. Most likely, her boobs will look incredibly unnatural at this stage.

This swelling happens because her body is pumping fluid into the space between her skin and the implants to help them heal. This makes the skin even tighter and makes her boobs look unnatural and feel tight and sore.

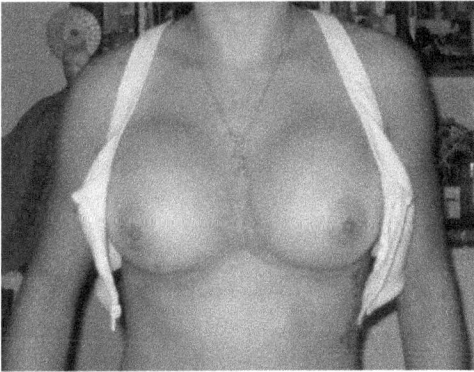

Jane on Day 2 post-op

Her boobs will feel very weird to her, and when she sees them, she will likely feel very emotional. They might not be quite what she wanted at this point, and they may freak her out.

There are a few things she can do to minimize the swelling. Make sure she is resting with her torso elevated. Doing this will help the swelling go down more than anything else. It may make her back sore, and she may complain or try laying flat. Also, taking bromelain pills can reduce the

> At first, the implants will feel too big and too high. DO NOT PANIC! This is normal. They will settle into place over the ensuing weeks. The surgeon will check for positioning at your woman's post-op visits to make sure her body is adapting well to the implants, that there is no sign of capsular contracture, and that the incisions are healing well.
>
> *Dr. Vip Says...*

swelling. Remind her to take it if her surgeon recommends it. Finally, don't forget to ice her boobs! It helps the body recover from the trauma and reduces swelling.

As for the height of her boobs, there's nothing you can do. Just accept that the law of gravity will keep working like it has for years. Her breasts will come down and look better as the skin and muscle stretch.

It's going to take several months (and up to a year in some cases) for her body to fully adjust to the implants and for them to look really good. Accept it. Know that every day that you see them high and tight is one day closer to fabulous boobs.

Jane knew what to expect after immense research, but still wasn't ready for how high and square-ish they looked and for how long they took to look better!

One of Jane's friends had a terrible experience. Her man didn't know what to expect and didn't know that her new breasts would be really high for the first few weeks after

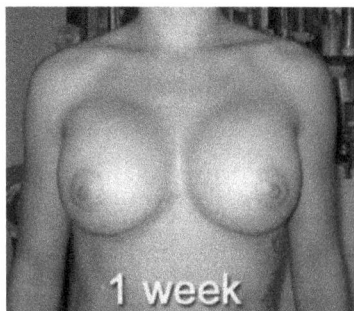

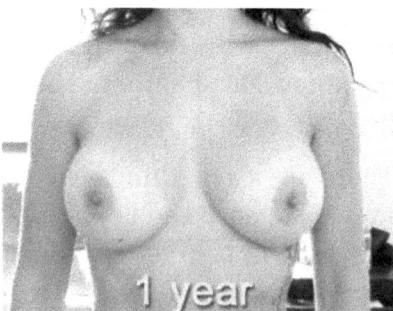

Over time they looked more natural

surgery. He insulted her breasts and said, "I can't look at you anymore!" This crushed her. Here she was, striving to be sexier, and he just killed her spirit. That's NOT how you win the game! Don't be that guy. Be sensitive to your woman's emotions.

Bruising

Her breasts may be bruised right after the surgery, or the bruises may develop a few days post-op. This is normal. Jane experienced minimal bruising, but varying degrees of bruising are normal.

The bruised areas may be extra tender, and she'll want them to fade.

To minimize the bruising she should take her arnica montana pills and apply arnica gel (if her surgeon recommends them).

See the section on "Protecting the Ball" to learn more about certain bruises you should look out for. Some of them can be signs of a serious complication.

Incisions

While they are probably covered by a surgical dressing, you might see her incisions. She will have incisions on either her breasts, armpits, or belly button. These can look nasty at first, so don't look if that kind of thing freaks you out.

These incisions are very painful fir her, so be understanding. The incisions are where infections are most likely to form. She needs to keep them clean, and you need to keep your hands away from them. Only touch the incisions if you are helping her clean them and using very clean hands.

> **Dr. Vip Says...**
>
> If your woman has any concerns about excessive discomfort, bleeding, or anything at all, she should call her surgeon's office. They will undoubtedly have an answering service to page the doctor. Other complications to look out for include redness around the incision site, clear drainage from the incision, opening of the incision, hardness of the implant, one side that is dramatically larger than the other, or difficulty breathing. If she has any concerns, it is always best to contact the surgeon and be seen immediately so that he can explain if what is happening is normal or not.

Mental Clarity

After surgery, the combination of anesthesia and pain medication may affect your woman's mental state. Most women feel groggy, sleepy, or a bit loopy, and may fall in and out of sleep.

A few women are so groggy that they say things that don't make much sense, or repeat the same things over and over. These women can have trouble remembering exactly what happened post-op. This "anesthesia amnesia" is exactly why you are in charge of her medication.

If she is bothered by her cloudy mind, remind her that she had anesthesia and is taking strong medication, and that it's expected that she be a little off-base. Tell her it's okay if she has some weird memories that come back in pieces.

Emotions

The entire breast augmentation process can be an emotional roller coaster. Be ready for mood swings and second-guessing. A combination of factors might throw her into a "what have I done?!" funk.

Between the anesthesia and pain medication's effects on her thinking, she can enter the "post-op blues", which may involve regret or guilt about getting implants.

She may also feel helpless and dependent on you or her caregiver. Most women are not used to being cared for hand and foot; they are usually the caregiver. This role reversal can be frustrating, especially if you aren't doing things exactly as she would.

Your woman will be anxious to see her new breasts will look like. She may worry that they are too big or too small, but she won't be able to tell because of the swelling. This uncertainty can be nerve-wracking.

Also, she wont be allowed to exercise for awhile post-surgery. So she won't have that outlet available to relieve stress. Added to this is the fact that she will be bloated after surgery. Being bloated plus not being able to work out can contribute to her depressed mood.

If she is a mother of a young child, she may be saddened by not being able to pick up, carry, or play with her child for a while.

So let's add up all of the factors affecting her. Anesthesia, drugs, bodily trauma, feelings of "buyer's remorse", helplessness, role-reversal, uncertainty, lack of exercise, bloating, and diminished ability to care for her children. No wonder she's acting strangely!

You know the best way to deal with your woman. So, I can't tell you precisely the best approach. Below are some guidelines to help you. You have to fill in the gaps appropriately for your specific case.

First, do your best to take care of her. Stay on top of the medication schedule, recording each time she takes a med. Keep her fed and hydrated, and help her to the bathroom as needed.

Walking is the best post-op treatment there is. Get your lady up to walk the evening of her procedure, even if it is just a short stroll around the house. Make sure you are there to help her if she gets dizzy—she probably won't, but it's better to be safe than sorry.

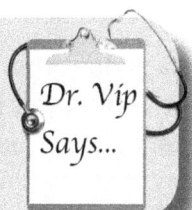

Dr. Vip Says...

For the first couple of days, you might have to help her shower once she feels she can stand. You may need to wash her hair for her for a while since she probably won't be able to lift her arms above her shoulders (especially if she got "unders"). Also, do all of the chores she included on the to-do list.

Do your best to help her, but don't try to be Superman. Do your best to help her, but don't try to be Superman. You will not do everything perfectly, but you can and should do your best. She may still complain, but I guarantee that she will appreciate all your effort and pay you back later.

The better she feels and the more positive she is, the faster she will heal, so give her compliments. She will know that she looks like crap, her hair is messed up, she has no make-up on and can't even sit up. But, by giving her a simple compliment, you can make her day. A lot of bad feelings can be melted away with a heartfelt compliment.

- "You're getting your color back in your skin."
- "You look happy, and your smile makes you look pretty."
- "Your boobs look better today!"

Any honest compliment will help her feel much better. They are worth their weight in gold!

Also, if she's still feeling down or upset about her condition, let her vent but remind her to be patient and that the process takes time. If she's like most women, your woman doesn't expect you to answer her concerns, but simply wants you to listen, let her know you understand, and show her you are there for her.

Each day after the first day, encourage her to walk around a little bit to get her blood flowing. This will help lift her spirits, help her heal, and take pressure off her back. She may try to do too much too soon, so encourage her to rest too.

Let her talk to you. Ask her how she's feeling—and without letting your mind wander to the score of the Vikings game—pay attention to what she says. Listening to her and responding appropriately will score you big points.

I recommend you try holding onto this trick for the rest of your relationship. Next time you ask her how her day was, really listen and show some interest. Many studies have shown that women find it sexy when a man listens to them!

You should do sweet things for her like brushing her hair or putting fresh sheets in her recovery area every couple of days.

You may also want or need to break out the big guns. Do things to make her feel pretty or buy her gifts. Jewelry, lingerie, gift cards for the spa, bath salts, gift certificates to Victoria's Secret or Amazon.com (or her favorite store) can really her feel awesome, forget about her pain, and think about how much she loves you. Win-win-win!

The most important thing for her emotions is to NEVER SAY ANYTHING NEGATIVE TO HER! Do not, UNDER ANY CIRCUMSTANCES, tell her her boobs look bad, even if she asks you point-blank. She knows what they look like. She's adjusting to them and the fact that they will change.

Weird Nipples

She may complain about her nipples. They may be ultra sensitive, burning, or sore. On the other hand, they may be completely numb. Or they could be a combination of both, shifting from one strange state to another. These sensations may be confusing and uncomfortable for her.

Remind her that this is normal, and that her nipples will heal and feel normal within 6-12 months.

If her nipples are extremely sensitive and uncomfortable, there are special silicone nipple covers that she can buy.

These can preventing her shirts, bras, and blankets from rubbing her the wrong way.

No matter what, keep your hands away from her nipples. Touching them now is a good way to get a slap in the face out of pure reflex.

"Boobie Farts"

In the first few days after surgery, you may hear some strange sounds coming from your woman's boobs. This is due to air that got trapped in her breast "pocket" when she was being sewn up.

You may hear a "gurgling" or "sloshing" sound. Don't worry, this is a normal part of the process and will not harm her, and will stop in two to four weeks when her body absorbs the air.

Wanting to Peek at Her Boobs

At this point, your woman probably doesn't want to show you her breasts.

Remember, she's in pain. She's on drugs and feels nauseous. She might be wrapped up in all kinds of dressings that constrict her breathing. She's got big foreign objects weighing down her chest. And her breasts probably look rather scary right now.

In other words, she's not going to be happy right now, so don't expect her to be flashing you her boobs yet.

Of course, after spending all this money, she is really going to want to look at her boobs too. Of course, you are dying to see them too.

A good surgeon will tell her (and you) how long she needs to keep her new sweater kittens wrapped up before peeking. Follow that advice. The doc knows what he's talking about. Help her resist the temptation to look too soon.

No Sex

As much as you are turned on by your woman having big new knockers (which are extra large right now due to the swelling), you need to be prepared to not get laid anytime soon.

Her body is recovering from surgery, so it her heart rate and blood pressure need to stay low. Also, any big movements can harm her breasts. SO NO SEX FOR NOW!

Her surgeon will tell her when it is safe for her to return (gradually) to fun time. Usually, surgeons recommend that she wait five or ten days. Some say two weeks. Some say three to six weeks. Listen to what he says.

If you're a guy with a high sex drive, get ready for a lot of cold showers and a invest in new bottle of hand lotion.

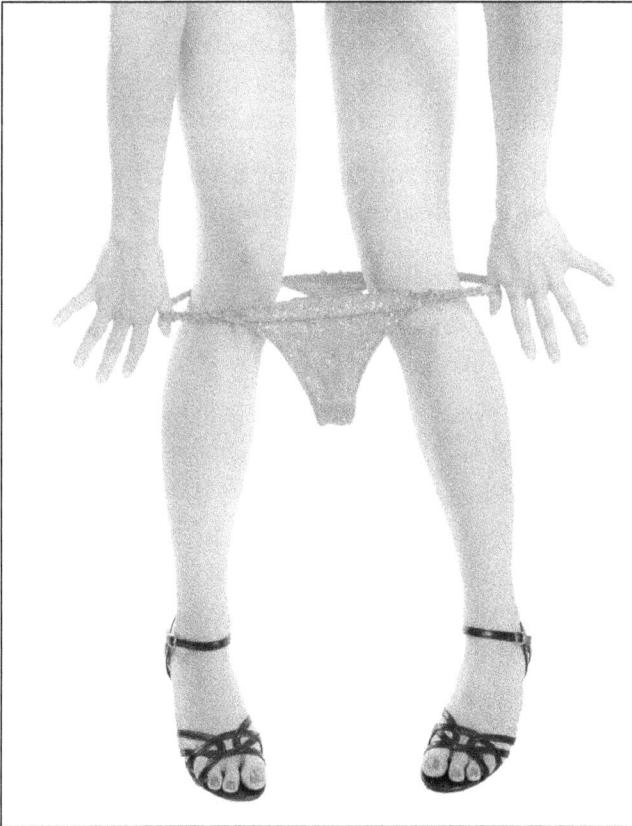

Protecting the Ball: Watching for Complications

Just like any good lineman, you need to have your head "on a swivel" to look out for any possible complications. You can run downfield, and block away defenders well before they get anywhere near stopping the touchdown!

Some complications are more likely a few weeks after the surgery, but some are likely to show up sooner.

If you play with "the girls" too soon after the surgery, there is a chance you can cause the incision to open up. Stitches can break, and this can ultimately lead to pain, infections, or nasty scars. If the incision is opening, have her contact her plastic surgeon immediately. And keep your damn hands off her breasts!

One thing to look out for is infections. If there is a LOT of redness, pain, strange-smelling drainage, or heat coming from near the incision, she may have an infection. If she has these symptoms or a fever, contact her surgeon right away.

Breast infections are rare (~1% of BAs), but as you may remember, Tom Brady's recovery from knee surgery was delayed by an infection. Infections not only lengthen the healing time, but—if left untreated—can spread and cause more severe complications. They are dangerous, but really easy to recognize and treat.

While almost every woman comes home with noticeable swelling and some bruising after her breast augmentation, there are a couple of complications that look like bruises but can be much worse.

A hematoma is a cavity that gets filled with blood. If she develops a VERY dark spot that gets swollen very fast (hours, not days) and hurts much worse than a bruise, she may have a hematoma.

In some cases these need to be surgically drained, but small ones can be absorbed by the body. If you think she has one, contact her plastic surgeon before you even take another breath.

Other fluids can collect in her body as well. A seroma is like a hematoma, but since it is not blood (just other body fluid), it won't get dark. This will be a painful area that swells quickly. This may need to be drained, so call the surgeon if you suspect one.

Post-Op Follow-Up Appointments

One great way to spot complications is to just let the pro do it.

Within the first 1-4 weeks after the operation, the surgeon should want your woman to come in to the office to see how her new boobs look.

If she has non-dissolving stitches in her body, he may remove them at this point. If your woman had pain pumps inserted they can come out at this time. The same is true of tubes used for draining TUBA incision tunnels.

The surgeon mostly wants to see how his work has turned out. He will be looking for any signs of complications that can slow her healing process, and to give her instructions on how to treat any complications that arise.

Surgeons do lots of follow-up after surgery to make sure everything is proceeding normally and to help calm women's fears. Most facilities and physicians call the patient the night of the surgery to make sure all is okay. Also, it's common that the surgeon will want to see your gal the day after surgery to make sure everything looks good. Then you're likely to drive her again for a postop weekly for four weeks, then every other week for a month.

Dr. Vip Says...

As she does her follow-up, you will notice that the breast implants descend on a weekly basis and even feel more natural as healing takes place. Many surgeons use sutures or stitches that absorb and just may have to cut the ends and not remove any sutures. Other surgeons, like me, use skin glue and have no sutures that need to be removed.

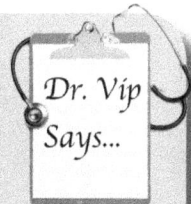

If there are any issues, the doc may have her come in multiple times within the first few weeks post-op.

Usually these follow-ups appointments are free. These are important for the surgeon to gauge her progress, recognize signs of complications, and answer her questions, so encourage her to go.

Congratulations!

After the first few days, you've made it through the roughest part of the recovery. Now you just need to be patient and know that those new boobs will look amazing soon enough!

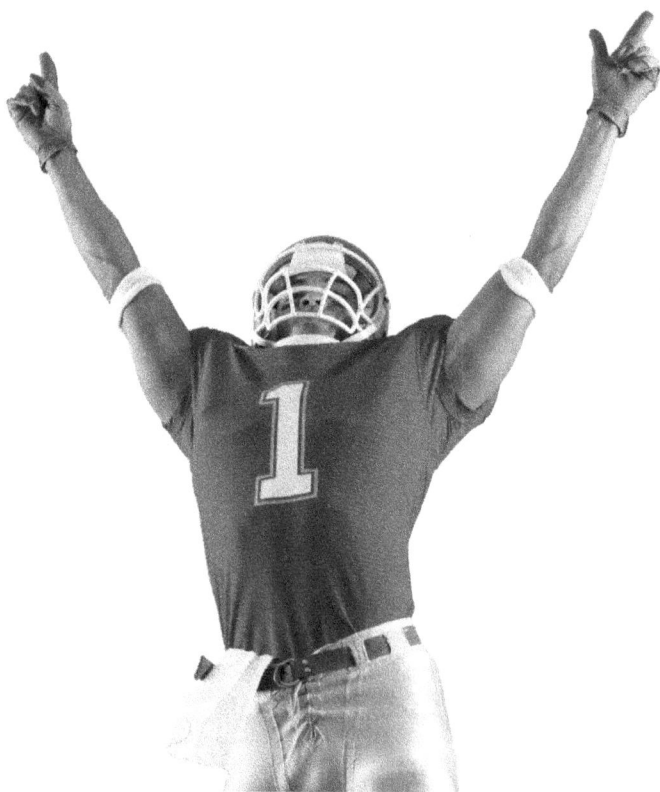

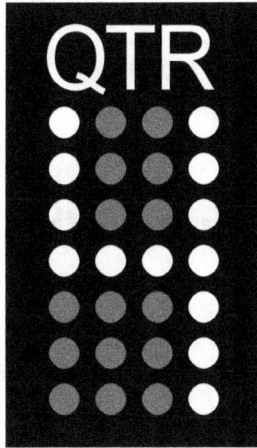

FOURTH
QUARTER:
PATIENCE

Questions this Section Answers:

How much longer do I have to WAIT to **see and play with her new boobs**?

When can I have sex with my now bustier woman?

What are the **physical symptoms of problems** we should look out for?

How can we **combat** the most common type of **complication**?

What if she starts to **regret getting the implants**?

What will it be like **when we go out** of the house together and what **should I be prepared** for?

How long will it take for her boobs to be completely ready?

* 17 *

A Long Way to Go

While the worst part of the recovery is typically the first few days post-op, it often takes a woman several weeks before she is healed. And once she is healed, it may then take several MONTHS before her body adjusts to the implants and her new breasts start to look *really* good.

That's right, MONTHS before her breasts are fully ready. That's not to say that they won't be bigger and more fun to play with and look at after week three. They just will not be completely settled into their final position for a while.

This will be a great way to learn patience.

During this time, the way you treat your woman and her new breasts can be important in determining how your relationship grows.

There are many new issues you will experience in the weeks after her surgery. These "firsts" and some potential psychological issues are discussed on the following pages.

Next, you'll learn how massaging your woman's boobs can be good for them... and very fun for you!

You'll also learn about the long, slow "drop and fluff" process that is like watching a receiver tightrope down the sideline and how "Pass Interference" could require a re-do of the surgery at any point.

Finally, we'll discuss what it really means to finally(!) cross the goal line and score the boobie touchdown. We'll finish with how to celebrate the TD and how to leverage it to improve your relationship.

18

The Breakaway: Weeks 2-4

Whenever a wide receiver catches a deep pass, three things can happen.

First, the defender could immediately tackle the receiver, push him out of bounds, or cause him to fumble.

The second option is for the receiver to run for a several yards before any of this happens to him.

The third—and most exciting—possibility is when the receiver is able to speed up, pull away from the defenders that are chasing him, and go all the way for the touchdown!

Wide receivers call it "the breakaway" when they break free of the defenders' reach and leave the cornerbacks and safeties diving at air.

Just as important as the catch is, the receiver has to be able to breakaway from the defense. Getting tackled immediately makes the catch meaningless.

In the "boobic play", getting over the initial recovery is the biggest hurdle, but by no means is it the end of the play. The extended recovery and the wait for her body to fully adjust to her implants is also vital to her final results.

Many "Firsts"

There are many firsts that you will both encounter in the weeks after her surgery. From looking and touching them, to sex and exercise, to seeing another man check her out when she's wearing a low-cut shirt, there will be many new experiences for you both.

The First Full View

Curiosity must have gotten the better of you by now, and I'm sure you've peeked at her boobs a time or two.

When you get your first real look at her boobs, try not to drool!

I hope you are really excited. I know I was when I got my first good look (without the surgical tape you see in the "Really High Beams" photo). The size was great, but because Jane got "unders", her boobs were still *very* high up and strangely shaped.

If your woman got "unders", her boobs may also look weird at first. There's nothing she can do about them now other than wait, so pointing out the flaws in her boobs will not help in any way. It can only hurt her psyche.

Even if your woman got "overs", chances are they won't look amazing yet.

Get a good look from the front, from the sides. Heck, even look at them from her point of view, and from "down below". Drink them in with your eyes!

Your job here is simple. SAY NOTHING BAD ABOUT HER BOOBS!

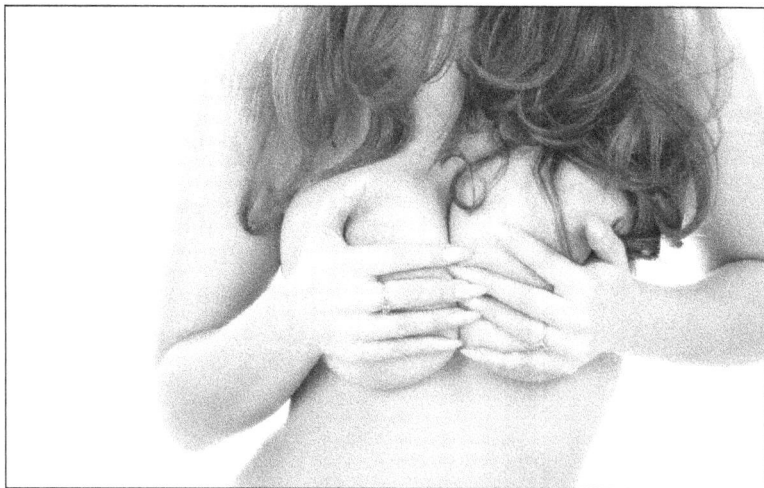

Tell her they look like a good size and that you are sure that they will look even better soon. Or, if they look good, tell her that!

She got the augmentation to feel better about herself, so help her feel good! If you mean it, tell her that you love them. Tell her how much they turn you on.

Ask her if she'd like you to take some pictures to compare to the "before" shots. This can lead to some fun like...

The First Touch

Your woman will probably be too swollen and sore from the surgery in the first week to even think about letting you really touch her breasts.

Only in the second week or so should you expect to get your first proper touches of her new boobs.

First, do not ask, beg, or plead to play with her boobies. She's in pain, and is probably barely touching them herself. She will let you touch them when she's ready.

Second, when she says she wants you to touch her breasts, ask her WHERE and HOW she wants you to touch them. She may have some areas that are still painful and will want you to steer clear of them.

Third, take it easy. You may be a big tough man, but you need to be gentle with her boobs. Many men are afraid of "ruining" her implants by doing something wrong. Like me, they fear subjecting her to the expenses and risks all over again, so they go extra gentle the first few times. This is a good thing.

Fourth, don't expect your first touches to be sexy at all. They will likely be very exploratory. You might poke a little or squeeze very lightly, but you will not be handling them like you would mid-coitus. You won't really be "playing with the twins" yet.

Finally, THEY WILL NOT FEEL LIKE NATURAL BREASTS AT THIS POINT! She probably still has fluid trapped in her breasts, and this may make them feel harder than normal until the swelling goes down. Time will fix this.

If your woman got "under the muscle" implants, then her pectoral muscles are probably still freaking out over the intruders stuck underneath them. Until her muscles fully relax to accept the implants, they will be very tight, and will make the upper part of her boob feel hard. Time will fix this also.

If your woman got silicone implants, they will probably end up (after time!) feeling just as good, if not better than real breasts. But not just yet. Again, time will fix this.

If your woman got saline implants, then you should remember that they will never fully feel like natural breasts (unless she had a lot of breast tissue to start). At this point, you will may begin to feel the difference between her implant and her breast tissue, but the swelling may cover it up. In the future, you will really be able to tell, as her breasts will be always be a bit firmer than real breasts. Time WILL NOT fix this.

The First Sex

Up to this point, your woman probably hasn't felt like having sex yet, and for good reason. She has been in pain, she needed to minimize boob movement, and she had to keep her heart rate and blood pressure low to keep from bursting blood vessels that can lead to hematoma. Most importantly, her surgeon told her to wait awhile before having sex, and she's listening to him.

You are probably thinking. "Dude, I just want to play with my new toys!" I was the same way. But you have to continue being patient.

You're not the only one with a sex drive. By now, your woman is probably dying for an orgasm too. But that doesn't mean it's a wild sex free-for-all.

She CAN NOT bounce around very much before her breasts adjust to the implants and heal, or she risks ruining the boob job. This means your first few sexual encounters with your newly enhanced woman must be relatively tame.

Play it *safe* and keep it *simple*.

Choose a position that is safe for her breasts and lets her remain relatively passive (to keep her heart rate low). Try simple missionary for the first few encounters post-op. Doggy-style can cause "the girls" to hang down and sway, and woman-on-top can cause a great deal of bouncing. These effects are not good.

Go SLOW, and pay attention to her.

Chances are good that you will both be nervous about this first intercourse post-op, and that's okay. Because of this, and because you both may be a little worried about harming her, you will both probably go extra gentle.

Also, it may be a good idea for her to keep her surgical bra or a sports bra on during the encounter to minimize un-

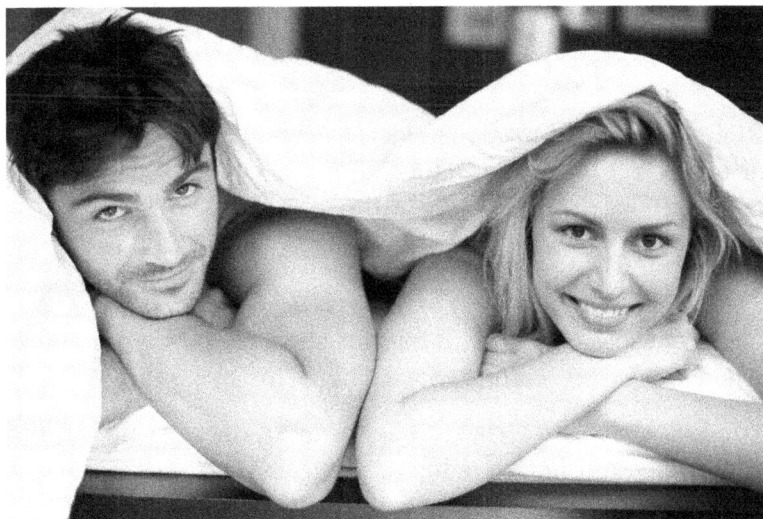

wanted boob bounce. It's not very sexy, but it's important for ensuring that her breasts look good for years to come.

Talk to her surgeon if you have any specific questions about sex. It may be a bit awkward to discuss, but he will give you good guidance.

Her First Exercise

Just like with sex, her surgeon has probably limited your woman's exercise post-op. Usually, she can begin light exercise two to four weeks after surgery, and start intense workouts at the gym or yoga studio after six or eight weeks.

Her ability to do upper body exercise may be limited for several months as her body adjusts to the implants.

Also, if she has "unders", your woman may notice her breasts move when she contracts her pectoral muscles. This is a normal part of having breast implants. Be ready, and don't make a big deal about it.

The First "What are You Wearing?!?" Moment

After going through the pain and expense of the surgery, your woman will likely have the urge to really show off her new toys.

Remember, most women's clothing is made to look nice with average or large boobs. The chances are high that there are many shirts that your woman has always wanted to wear, but she never thought she would look good in them... until now.

Some of these clothes will be a lot more revealing than what you are used to seeing her wearing. This may startle you.

You know she has a right to be proud of her new figure, but you don't want her showing it all off to everyone!

You can't order her to cover them up. You can tell her that it makes you uncomfortable and ask her to change clothes. However, accept that she will wear what she wants to wear from now on and chances are it's going to be something sexy.

Sometimes women want to wear a top that's really revealing before their breasts have had time to heal. This can be to the point where it doesn't look good.

Jane went on a shopping rampage and bought lots of low-cut shirts, and wore them exclusively for the first few weeks. Many of them looked good on her, but in a few her breasts looked VERY OBVIOUSLY fake and not-so-attractive.

This is where I said, "WHAT are you wearing!?"

I didn't do a good job of expressing that her boobs didn't look as good in that shirt as she thought. She interpreted my requests to cover up as insecurity about her flaunting her boobs. I wish I had been able to say it better. Learn from my mistake!

If you find your woman is wearing something way too revealing too soon, let her know, but be honest. Say, "I know it may seem like I'm being insecure about your new sexiness, but I am just trying to be honest. That's a sexy shirt you have on, and I bet it will look a lot better once your breasts aren't as swollen or high up. Until then, would it make more sense to change into something else?"

Good luck with that. I hope you do better than I did.

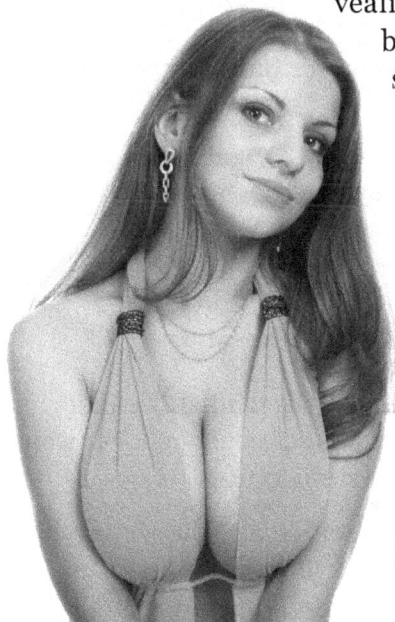

The First Stares

Chances are that her larger breasts will attract attention. You'll probably notice more guys checking her out. You might even catch some ladies checking her out.

This might make your woman feel special. She's a girl, so she *probably* likes attention (What a sexist statement!). She may like it as she gets flirted with more frequently due to her bigger breasts.

But don't worry about losing her; you're the man with the hottie!

Everyone is going to look at you and think you're a major stud to get a girl like that. Other men will wonder what you have that they don't. You can just smile.

Remember, you're the one with her. She is WITH YOU! Others may catch a glimpse of her figure. They'll just be jealous of you because you get to go play with the "treasure chest".

If you are in a good relationship with your woman, and you have helped her throughout this journey, she will have no reason to be interested in what other guys and girls think. She will like the attention but never have any intention of doing anything with them.

You should remain confident and be proud of the man you are. You deserve to enjoy those "flesh melons" and she knows it!

Her First Post-Op Dentist Appointment

Many people are afraid of going to the dentist. Dentists use sharp tools. For most people this is scary enough. For women with implants, there can be more to fear.

The sharp tools that dentists use can make abrasions on the teeth and gums. Germs can sneak into these abrasions, and cause simple infections. Usually, the human body will fight such infections off. The body's automatic response to infection is to protect the body from foreign invaders (breast implants, pacemakers, or screws), and this can cause complications.

That means dental work can cause boobie problems! Bet you never thought about THAT when she told you she wanted a boob job!

Many surgeons recommend that women who have implants take antibiotics prior to all dental visits. So prior to your woman's first dental visit post-op, remind her to call her surgeon, and he will probably give her a prescription for a large "loading" dose to take before she sees the dentist. While many surgeons recommend this for all dental visits, some only give antibiotics for the first one or two visits.

Post-Op Psychological Issues

"Buyer's Remorse"

Have you ever felt "buyer's remorse" after picking up a cool new toy or spending more than you had planned on a new suit? You might wonder whether the item you just got was worth the price you paid.

Well, your woman may experience strong "buyer's remorse" with her implants. Not only did they cost a lot in terms of time and money, but they may also still feel uncomfortable. This is makes the "buyer's remorse" all the worse.

"Buyer's remorse" can be especially strong among women who don't think their surgeon gave them exactly what they wanted.

Some women wish they had never had the surgery, and others wish they had made different implant choices.

If your woman experiences "buyer's remorse", there's not that much you can do. Remind her that her breasts will look better soon enough and that if she wants to change them down the road, that you two will talk about it. Break out the "Reminders to Herself" sheet if need be.

"Boobie Greed"

One particular type of post-augmentation "buyer's remorse" is "boobie greed", in which the woman regrets not having gotten larger implants. This can kick in immediately or months post-op.

A lot of women who get implants started with small to average sized breasts and wanted to feel average or a little bigger than average.

After the swelling is over, and they are getting out of the house more, some women realize that their implants have not given them the size and shape they had in mind. Others just get used to the swollen size, and are disappointed after the swelling goes down.

Some women will talk non-stop about this. They will complain about not getting bigger implants for the amount of time, money, and pain they invested.

They may notice women with very large breasts and comment on them. Some women will just complain about a specific aspect of their boobs that they wish were different. "I wish I had better cleavage." "Why didn't I get a double D?" "I wish I had more side-boob!".

Most women will grow to accept their new breasts and realize how much of an improvement they are over their original pair. The little imperfections will be forgotten.

Other women, however, will let "boobie greed" consume their thoughts. They want bigger breasts, and they want them yesterday! These women are often willing to have another surgery almost immediately to get bigger implants.

"Boobie greed" is a very real post-augmentation psychological issue. If your woman is experiencing it, there are a couple of things you can do. First, remind her how much of an improvement what she has now is over what she had before. Tell her how beautiful she is and how her new breasts contribute to that. Again, break out the "Reminders to Herself" worksheet if need be.

Also, remind her that her body is still adjusting to her implants, and that she will mentally get used to them too. Once she's had time to become accustomed to her breasts and has talked with women who got much bigger implants, she may reconsider.

Basically, you should ask her to give her breasts a real opportunity to make her happy before deciding she needs new ones. Also, most surgeons won't give a woman a redo to bigger implants before 6-12 months post-op, so she likely can't do anything about it anyway.

Ball Protection: Watching for Complications

Keep a look out for these complications.

Symmastia (aka "Uni-Boob")

Sometimes, in an effort to give your woman the best cleavage possible, the surgeon will make the "pocket" of each breast too close to the cleavage line. When this happens, the muscle and skin can lift in the middle and allow the implants to touch, leaving no space between the breasts.

The surgeons call this "symmastia" but it's often dubbed "uni-boob" (like a hairy man's uni-brow). This is not common, and is almost always due to surgical error or choosing implants too wide for a given woman's chest. If this happens, it can usually only be fixed with another surgery, but some surgeons recommend using a special "thong bra" that forces the breasts apart.

This usually does not show up until a couple of weeks or months after the operation, but can happen immediately in some cases.

Bottoming Out

We discussed the "pocket" where the surgeon puts the implants. Sometimes, the bottom of this skin "pocket" pulls away from the muscles and ribcage under the weight of the implant. The implant then slips down under the skin, further south than it should.

This is not likely to happen, but the result is bad. It's visually undesirable and can be uncomfortable for the woman. The better the surgeon, the less likely this is to happen. Better surgeons will make the right recommendations based on the thickness of her skin and muscle.

Close cousins of "bottoming out" are "double-bubble" and "snoopy boob", in which the implant and breast tissue seem to be two separate things.

In the rare case that any of these should happen, you both will notice that her breasts look odd. She should contact her surgeon immediately, and revision surgery is likely.

Weird Sensations

She may still be experiencing weird sensations in her breasts and especially over her nipples. Strange tingling is common in this time period as the nerves start fixing themselves. Be gentle and don't touch her nipples too much. They may still likely feel raw and painful, totally numb, or somewhere in between. There's nothing to do about it, other than give it time and stay away as much as she asks!

Capsular Contracture

Do you know how an oyster makes a pearl?

When a single grain of sand enters an oyster, it is abrasive to the inside of the oyster. So the oyster lets out some fluid around the grain of sand, which hardens to make it less rough and annoying. It does this again and again, laying multiple layers of hard shell around the sand. Eventually, it builds up to a nice big pearl that's almost totally smooth.

As a defense mechanism, your body will form a layer of scar tissue around any intruding foreign body. I had a cool example with a piece of auto glass that was stuck in my hand for 10 months. Every few weeks, the glass would break out of its scar tissue shell (usually when I was carrying something heavy or hitting a softball) and cut the inside of my hand. After a week or so, a new shell of scar tissue formed. This continuous pattern was a real annoyance.

Even something less 'shard of glass'-like —such as a breast implant— will cause her body to react with a layer of scar tissue totally surrounding the implant. Usually, this scar tissue stays fairly soft and pliable. For many **possible** reasons but no **one known** cause, this scar tissue can harden and contract over time.

The fibers within this scar tissue start to pull together, putting a great deal of pressure on the implant. Since saline and silicone are not very compressible, the implant just ends up getting very hard. This makes her

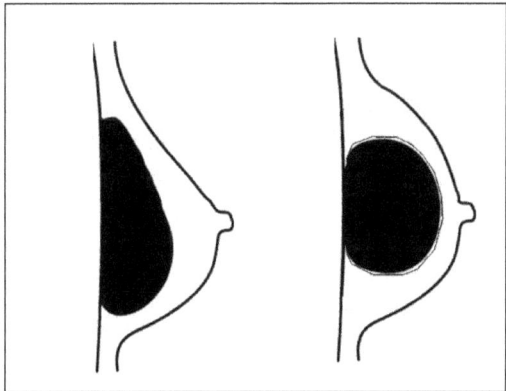

Capsular contracture squeezes the implant into a rounded shape, getting hard and looking strange.

> Statistically speaking, capsular contracture and implant failure are the most common risks of breast implant surgery. When a breast implant is inserted, as with any kind of foreign material, the body will create a shell or capsule around it. This is normal and natural. This shell is made of fibrous tissue and can shrink a bit over time. If it shrinks too much, it can compress the implant, causing it to feel hard and look strange. This can become painful and may eventually require that the implant be removed. Most women replace implants after a serious case of capsular contracture, although some women choose not to do so.
>
> *Dr. Vip Says...*

boobs feel very firm and look round or misshapen. It can be accompanied by a dull ache.

This strange scar-tissue process is called "capsular contracture" (or "CC" for short), and is the most common complication resulting from breast enlargement surgery. It can happen anytime from a few weeks after to years down the road.

Neither of you want this! It can lead to breasts that are as hard as wood or create a really bad 'bolted on grapefruit' look.

Keep an eye out for CC. If it's bad enough, surgery may be needed to cut the scar capsules.

Some surgeons think that certain medications can help prevent and/or fix CC, along with physical manipulation of the breast.

Jane actually had a mild case of capsular contracture and was prescribed a homeopathic supplement called "Scar Formula Multiplex", which is available at several online pharmacies.

The Multiplex comes as little tiny balls about the size of BBs. Every 1-2 hours she would put 4 of these sweet-tasting white BBs under her tongue until they dissolved. She kept this up for six months! These supplements are usually used for a minimum of three weeks, but work best as a long-term treatment used to dissolve scar tissue

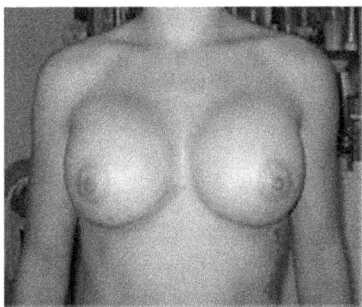 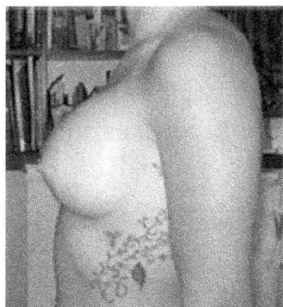

One Week

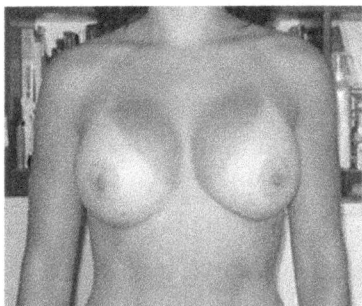 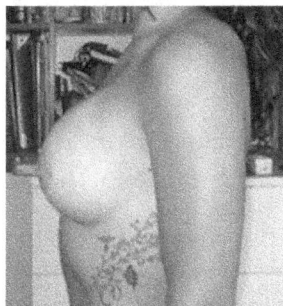

Three Months

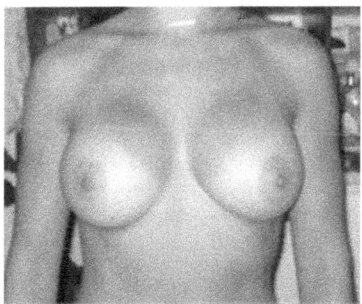 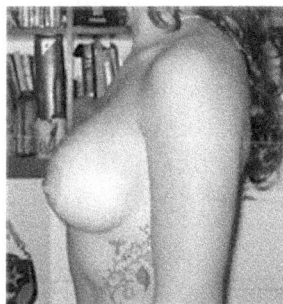

Six Months

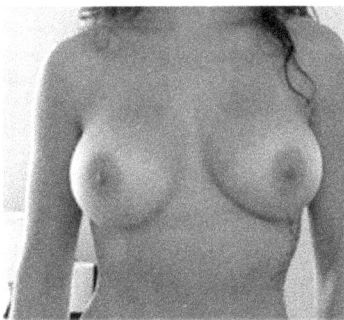 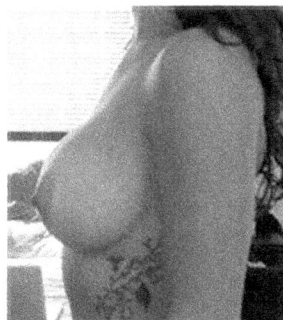

One Year

Yes this was a real annoyance to her, but it never tasted bad, and it did help her overcome her CC. There are no scientific research studies proving that it works or works any better than other treatment methods, but it did work for Jane. Judge for yourselves if you think it's worth a shot.

If your woman develops capsular contracture, she should contact her surgeon about her treatment options.

Downfield Blocking: Boob Massage!

One of the best things a lineman can do to help out a receiver running for a touchdown is to run downfield and block the defenders. Even if a defender is already far away from the receiver, the farther away, the better.

In order to keep your ugly opponent, CC, from halting your boobie touchdown, some surgeons believe massaging the breasts keeps everything soft.

You don't have to wait for your woman to develop CC to start the massaging. Some doctors say it can prevent it from happening in the first place.

On the other hand, some surgeons think that massage causes inflammation which can lead to CC. She should follow her surgeon's instructions.

Jane was proactive and started massaging her breasts before she found out she had CC. Her doctor showed her several massage techniques at her request, and she began them 3 days post-op.

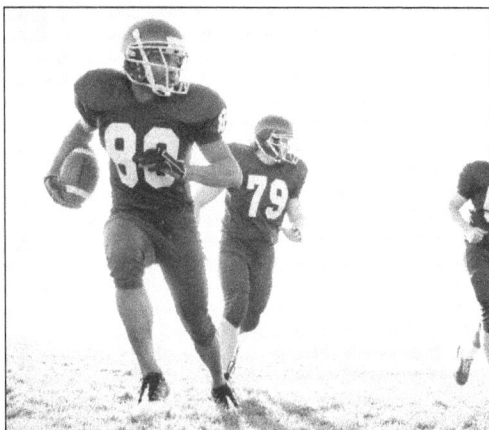

It was "too bad" (my words) that she couldn't do all the techniques from the proper angles by herself. It also was "too bad" that her hands got tired very easily.

What was she to do? She did what made the most sense. She asked me help to help massage her boobs!

You can imagine what a pain, what a chore it is to HAVE spend ten minutes a day massaging your woman's big, new, beautiful breasts!

It was wonderful. It was my favorite part of the day. I've never liked following "doctor's orders" quite so much.

Your woman's surgeon may recommend that she have you massage her breasts. Or he may just tell her that it's not going to harm her for you to do it. Unless the surgeon specifically says, "don't massage her mammaries", you should jump at the chance to have fun and help her out.

By the time you get to the point where the surgeon asks you to massage her boobs, you'll probably be dying to play with them anyway. I know I was!

Massaging her new boobs will help to loosen her muscles and cause her boobs to get softer. It will also help you grow accustomed to how her new breasts look and feel. And it may get the two of you in the mood. ;)

The goal of the massage is to move the implant around in the pocket and to put pressure on it so that the scar tissue around it stays soft and flexible.

To do this, use your hand to push the implants around in the pocket. You can push them up towards her shoulders, in to make more cleavage, and down toward the bottom of her boobs. NEVER PUSH HER IMPLANTS OUT TOWARD HER SIDES! Doing so can hurt her chances of having good cleavage (which most women want) by causing her implants to slowly move outward.

The first few times I tried massaging her boobs, I went very easy on them because I thought they were fragile. After talking with her surgeon, I realized that they were really tough and I could really manhandle them!

Seriously, breast implants are strong. You are not going to pop them. Give them a good squeeze. Your woman will be in pain long before you damage the implants.

Another great massage method is to just squeeze each boob and play with it however you want... without hurting your woman of course.

I really liked getting some lotion and massaging that into her boobs (making sure to not touch ANYWHERE near her incisions until they were fully healed).

Passive Solo Massage

In addition to the massage, Jane liked to keep additional pressure on the implant for extended periods of time to stretch the scar tissue of her capsular contracture.

She would lay down on a large hardcover book for about an hour each night (with her weight resting on one or both implants). She usually did this while shopping/chatting on the internet or while watching TV or movies.

So, if you can't or don't want to massage her boobs, then this is an alternative that may help soften her new boobs.

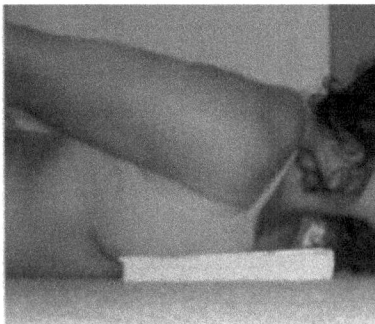

Flat on both boobs   *One boob at a time*

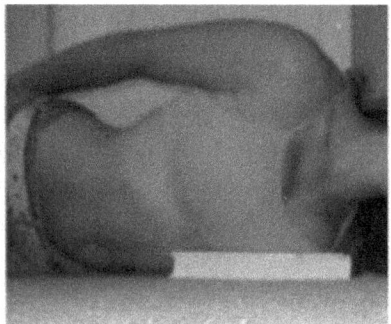

* 19 *

Tightroping the Sideline:
Time Slows Down

Often as a receiver take the final steps to the goal line, he streaks down the sideline. He runs as if on a tight-rope, keeping himself as far away from the defenders as possible. As the excitement builds– "Will he make it or not?"– time seems to slow down.

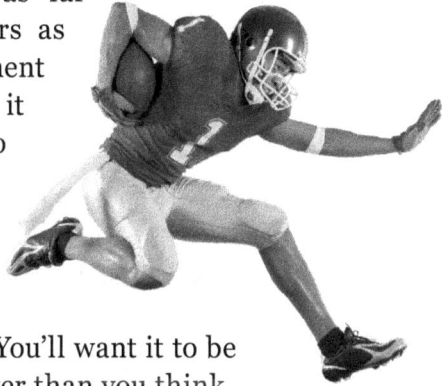

As you get closer to the boobie touchdown, it may seem like time is moving in slow motion. You'll want it to be over, but it will take longer than you think.

I've had two sports-related surgeries that required me to get screws put in my body. Each time, it took a long time for my body to grow accustomed to these foreign objects. It was nearly ten months before I really felt like my body parts were mine again.

Your woman's body will take a long time to get used to the implants, which are WAY bigger than the screws I had put into my knee and shoulder.

If you haven't gotten the message yet, the game plan for guys is **Patience, Patience, Patience**.

All you can do is wait and let her boobs get better with time. Between six months and one year after surgery is when most women's breasts start to look like and feel like natural breasts. Depending on how the surgery was performed and how tight your woman's skin and muscles are, it may take up to a full year.

During this long period of her boob improvement, there are several things you may notice along the way.

First her boobs will stop being up near her chin and will slowly start to lower to a more normal height. Sometimes, implants will drop at different rates. She may be uneven for a bit, but this is usually nothing to worry about. They will even out in time.

Another big event in the months after the augmentation is the return of normal nipple sensation.

Nine months after surgery , Jane started getting feeling back in her nipples. They grew to become more sensitive than they were before the surgery (in a good way).

If your woman gets a lot of pleasure from her nipples and is frustrated that they don't feel the same as before, reassure her that it should work itself out within the first year.

Finally, in the months following her surgery, her surgical scars should start to fade.

Depending on the incision location your woman chose, she may have some visible scarring from the surgery. As time goes by, the scars should get lighter, softer, and less noticeable. Being disciplined in applying various ointments and silicone sheets can help make scars disappear faster, but her surgeon should tell her exactly what to use.

All surgeons agree that *time* and keeping scars *out of the sun* are the biggest factors in making scars go away fast. They tend to disagree on everything else.

Many surgeons think that applying Steri-Strips after the sutures are removed helps incisions heal best. To reduce scarring, some surgeons recommend medications such as Mederma, which requires multiple applications per day for several weeks. Others recommend special sheets of medicated rubber called "silicone sheets", "scar sheets", or "scar guard" to make scars disappear faster.

* 20 *

Crossing the Goal Line: Boobs Finally Settle

Have you ever bought new bed pillows? Or have you been at home when your woman brought some home? Most pillows come shrink-wrapped in plastic so that they are compressed a little. If you squeeze it while wrapped up, it will not feel soft.

Well, if you take a fork and puncture the plastic in a few places, the plastic will weaken. As air rushes in through the holes, the pillow expands and stretches the plastic.

If you touch the pillow now, it will feel more like what you want under you head at night.

The pillow will continue to get softer and fluffier. With more holes, the plastic will relax more and the pillow will fluff to its full capacity.

A woman with "unders" will experience something like this as her breasts "fluff".

As her skin and pectorals stretch to accommodate the implant, her breasts will slowly start to feel softer. After what seems like a million years, but is really only a few months, they will become softer and look more natural. The implants will take on a less "round" shape and she'll have a better slope to the top of her breast. This is the "drop".

For women who get subglandular breast augmentation ("overs"), it is a much more straightforward process. Since the muscles don't need to stretch, the breast implants will settle into place within a few months. Of course, the implants don't really move; the implant filler moves to the lower part of the implant as the skin stretches to accommodate the implant as they "settle".

Implant Drop/Fluff Transition

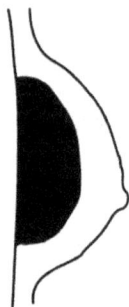

Post-Surgical Breast

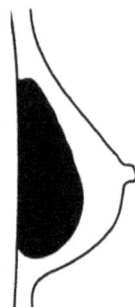

Dropped & Fluffed Breast

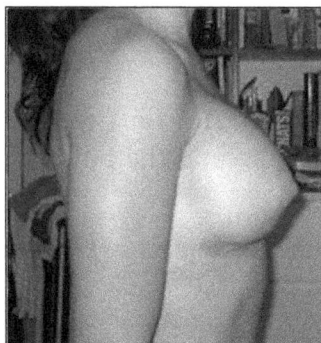

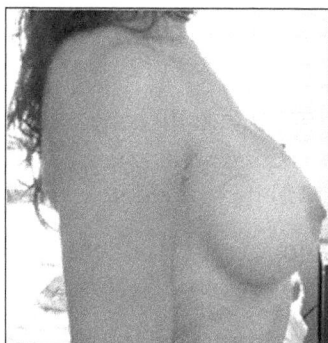

In the early weeks, the implants are compressed by muscle and/or skin and breast tissue, which causes the breasts to be more full above the nipples in the upper pole. The nipples may point slightly downwards and the breasts may lack fullness and roundness at the bottom. They can appear flat or square in shape. New implants usually don't fill out bras quite right, and can be hard and firm for several weeks/months.

When the implants "drop," they don't actually go anywhere. As the muscles and tissues stretch around the implant, the substance inside the implant shell (silicone or saline) responds to gravity by sliding down toward the bottom of the bag. The result is a more natural looking breast that is fuller at the bottom and behind the nipple. At this stage they get soft, squishy and more moveable.

Once your woman's breasts have "settled" or "dropped and fluffed", then you are there! You have scored the boobie touchdown!

Offensive Pass Interference: Revision Surgery

If at any point, your doctor realizes that something has gone wrong either in surgery or in the recovery phase, he may suggest that your woman get "revision surgery". This means she needs a "do-over" to fix something.

The need for revision surgery is always a possibility. You should be prepared for this scenario. Some doctors perform revision surgery for free, others charge only operating room and anesthesia fees, while some will charge just as much as the first surgery. This is something to consider when choosing a surgeon.

You can think of a revision just like an offensive pass interference was called on your previous deep pass. Sure, you lost a few yards, but you can try the same deep pass play again. You WILL score that touchdown!

As we've discussed, over time your woman may start to wish her breasts looked a little different even after her surgery. She may want bigger or smaller implants or wish she had a different profile. With this desire, she may **choose** to have a "re-do", which is different from revision surgery because it is voluntary.

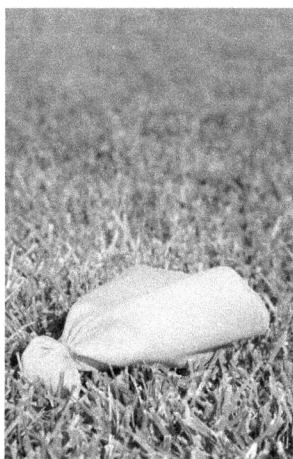

Be ready, she might want to talk about a re-do! And of course, there's always the chance that she will need to get her implants replaced 10, 20, or 30 years down the line even if everything goes perfectly.

Big High Five!: Celebrate the TD

Congrats! You've had lots of patience and are ready to reap the benefits of your woman having brand new breasts.

Finally! It seems like it has been going in slow motion, right?

Her breasts are finally ready. They have fully "dropped and fluffed" or "settled" and are now at their best.

Her breasts now look more natural because her body has adjusted to her implants, and they now sit a little lower. No more boobs in her chin!

Let the fun begin!

Are you excited to get to look at her new knockers? You get to see her boobs up close. It's wonderful.

Hell, just looking at them near your face isn't all that matters. It's really nice to see your woman approaching you from across the room when she has fabulous breasts.

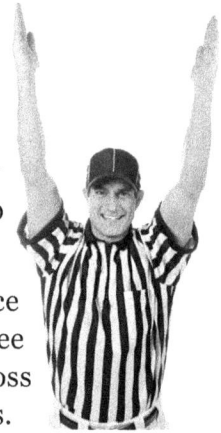

More importantly, during this process, your woman has been able to overcome what she saw as a flaw. She will feel more confident as a result of looking the way she wants.

More confidence means that she will feel sexier. When she feels sexier, she will want you more.

Be happy about what you've been through. Smile and be a friend and lover to your woman. It's worth all the time and effort just to be able to enjoy her boobs now and for many years to come!

Now that her boobs are settled, you can take some sexy photos or buy her some more sexy bras and tops to celebrate. Maybe now is a good time for that trip to Hawaii you've always talked about...

* 21 *
Second Half Momentum

When a team scores a touchdown right before half-time, momentum tends to shift in their direction. In the second half of the game, they can come out strong and win against tough opponents.

Well, you have just completed your pass and have scored an amazing boobie touchdown! Congratulations!

No matter what your relationship was like before her surgery, you can use the momentum from this boobie touchdown to help the rest of your relationship.

Not only has this touchdown changed your woman's body, self-image, and attitude, but hopefully it has also improved aspects of your relationship as you've connected more.

If you followed the advice in this book, you have probably talked a lot with your woman and grew to understand her a little bit better. You have taken care of her by doing nice things for her and maybe buying her little gifts.

Keep doing these things in the future and see how your relationship thrives.

Talk to your woman more. Ask her about her day and her interests, and really listen to her. This will take a little of your time, but it will help to make your relationship stronger. Of course, thoughtful gifts and helping out around the house will also make you both happier.

These simple acts can get you more lovin' from your lady, and keep her thinking of no one but you even though she's getting more attention from other men.

Leverage your momentum and carry it through to the rest of your relationship! Use it to help you win the game of life!

Victory In The Game Of Life
Is Up To You!

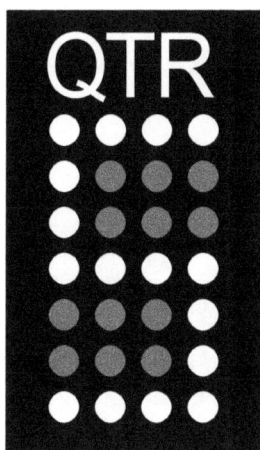

POST-GAME: EPILOGUE

Questions this Section Answers:

How are Jane and Dallas doing now?

Did Jane get another surgery?

* 22 *

Conclusion

Learning and Growing

Going through the breast augmentation process with Jane was great, and it drew us closer to each other.

It also taught us each a little more about ourselves. I learned how to be patient, and I learned how much I like large breasts.

As we continued learning more about ourselves, we realized that we really weren't the right match for one another. About two years after her surgery, we mutually decided to end our relationship.

We realized that things weren't going to work for us in the long term, and we ended it before things got too far along. We had never seriously discussed marriage and children, and considering how many years we were together, that fact was strange. As sad as it was, we had to acknowledge that we were not the ones that would make each other happy for the rest of our respective lives.

So, Jane and I didn't last. However, we both see it as for the best. She didn't leave me and I didn't run from her.

Jane is still a great friend of mine, and I care for her deeply. Her help on this book was unbelievable. I couldn't have written it without her.

Jane's Surgeries

After Jane's breasts had healed and she gained confidence, she began exercising much more. She started lifting weights, doing Pilates, and practicing yoga. She lost some weight and her body got a lot tighter.

As is the case with all women, when she lost the weight, some of it came from her breasts. Since she didn't have all that much natural breast tissue to start with, every bit that she lost brought her implants that much closer to the skin.

We both began to notice her breasts showing more ripples, especially when she bent over. Although I was okay with it, this bugged her.

We could also feel the difference. Her implants became very obvious to the touch. I didn't love this, but I never complained. She felt that it was a big deal.

Also, her implants had migrated away from the center of her chest a bit. Whether this was from the very rounded shape of her rib cage, the movement of her pectorals from increased exercise, or just her body's reaction to the implants, her cleavage was reduced. She didn't like that.

After weighing her options, Jane chose to get a new set of implants. Since she had seen many many examples of his work, she felt comfortable choosing to go with the same surgeon.

She chose silicone implants for a more natural feel. She chose a periareolar incision, knowing that he would give her little to no scarring. Since her muscles were already stretched, she again went with under the muscle placement.

She really wanted to have more cleavage after this second surgery, so she elected to use slightly larger implants. After discussing it with the surgeon, she also requested that he move the pocket in further and put a couple of dissolvable stitches on the outside edge of her breasts.

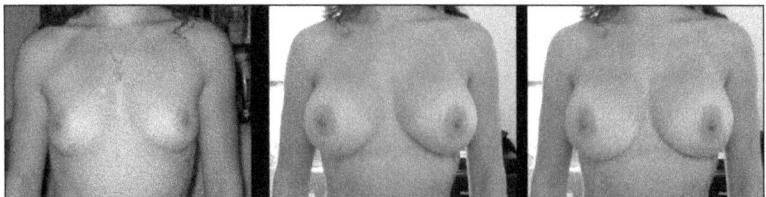

Before   **After 1st (350 cc)**   **After 2nd (500 cc)**

Jane was initially very happy with her new breasts. She achieved the increased cleavage she sought, and the feel was very natural.

However, after awhile, she began to realize that the new implants were just a little too big for her frame. She admitted that she got greedy and wanted to warn women not to make the same mistake she did.

She has also experienced a few other issues related to changing sizes, such as ripples on the inner cleavage and increased muscle flex distortion.

She said that if she had it to do over again, she wouldn't have had the surgery or would have switched to silicone without changing the size of her implants.

Also, between her breast surgeries, Jane also got a nose job (rhinoplasty). She got her nose reduced slightly. It looks great.

Some women do find more things to fix after their first surgery. Be ware!

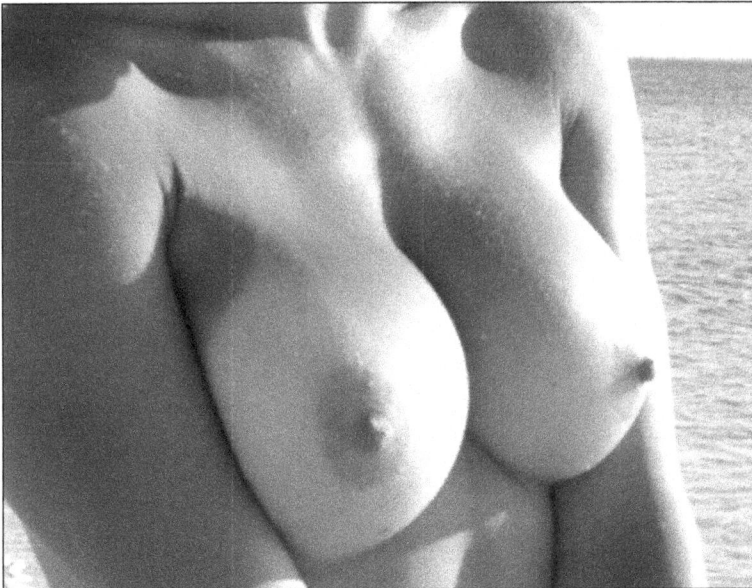

* 23 *

Coach Dallas's Final Thoughts

Why are you still reading? Get out there and play with those boobs!

Ok, I'll assume she's in the bathroom or something, so here's a few final thoughts.

You are to be congratulated for taking the time to read a book to better understand your lady as she makes changes in her life. Good for you!

I hope you have a great number of years enjoying those new bigger breasts!

Treat her well and love her. Be a man; be great to your woman. Win the game of life!

I hope that my book has helped you as your woman decided about and went through with breast augmentation. I know I wish I had someone to help me through the process.

Please let me know if this book was helpful to you so I can help more men. Did you think it was great? Did you think it was all BS? Were you confused because you don't even know what a football is? Whatever the case, let me know by emailing me at
Dallas@FootballAndBoobs.com

I'm always interested to learn about other men's perspectives and experiences with breast augmentation. Other men could learn a lot from what you have to say.

In fact, I'm so curious to hear your story, that I've set up a special email account for it. You can send me your story at

Touchdown@FootballAndBoobs.com

If you are willing, I might choose to share your story so that we can help other men find hooter happiness!

APPENDIX:

Dr. Vip Dev's Surgical Examples

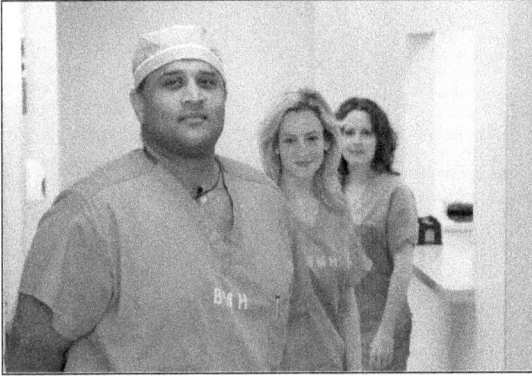

Dr. Vip Dev and his team perform hundreds of breast augmentations each year.

Following are sets of before-and-after photos of women that Dr. Dev has operated on. Also included are some bad surgical results from other surgeons that he was asked to repair.

Breast Augmentation Examples

Patient 1 started with small breasts and got a noticeable increase in breast size. These are saline implants put in through a periareolar incision (around the nipple).

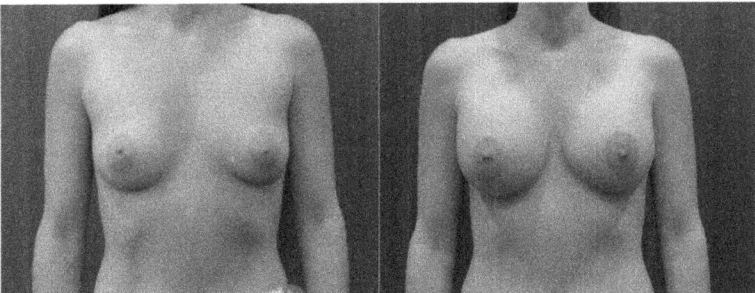

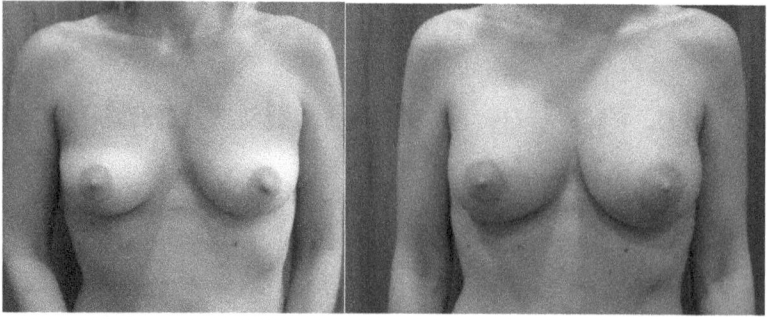

Patient 2 started with small breasts and got a subtle increase in breast size. These are silicone implants put in through a periareolar incision (around the nipple).

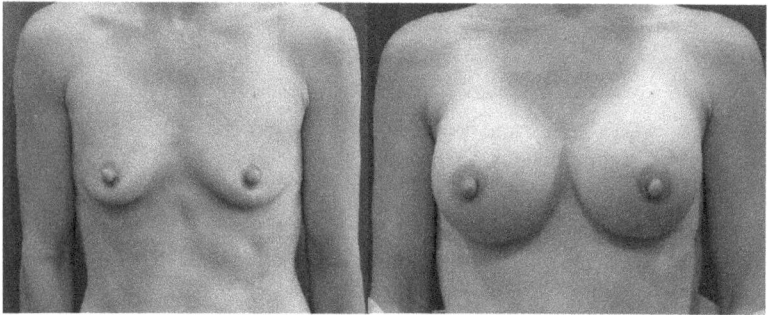

Patient 3 started with very small yet droopy breasts and got a very noticeable increase in breast size. These are saline implants put in through a periareolar incision (around the nipple).

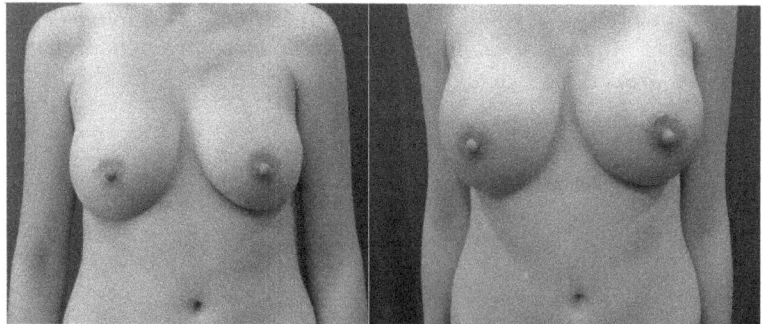

Patient 4 started with large breasts and got a subtle increase in breast size. These are silicone implants put in through a periareolar incision (around the nipple).

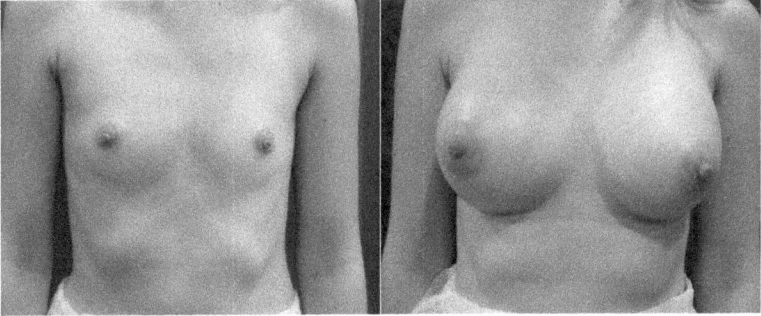

Patient 5 started with very small breasts and got a very noticeable increase in breast size. These are saline implants put in through a periareolar incision (around the nipple).

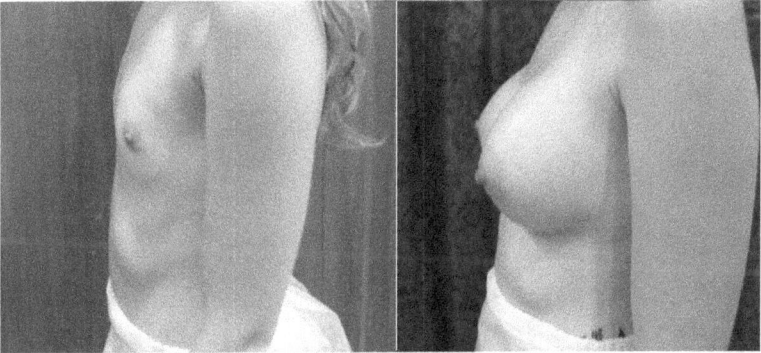

Examples of Other Types of Breast Surgery

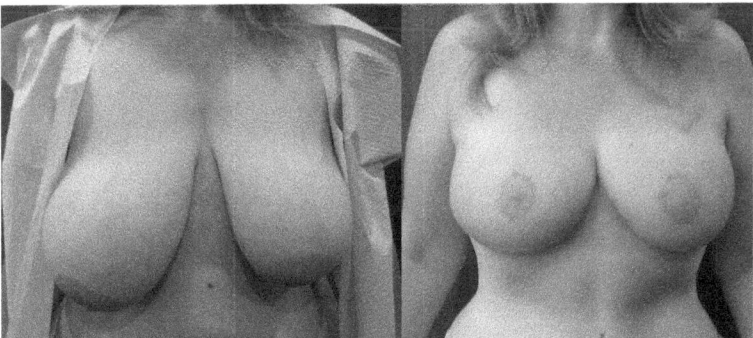

Patient 6 started with very large, droopy, uneven breasts and got a reduction in breast size. The technique Dr. Vip used did not leave her with a large vertical scar, as many surgeons do.

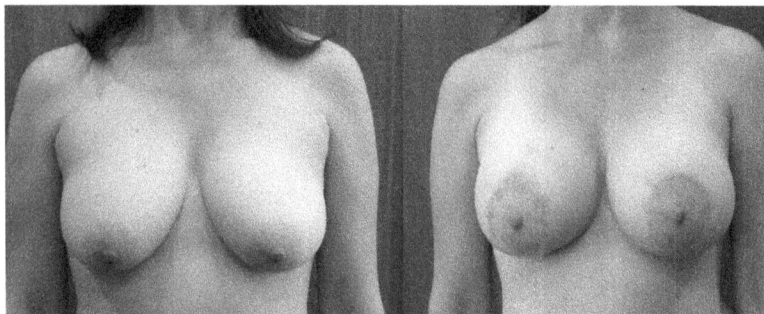

Patient 7 started with large, droopy breasts and got both a breast lift and breast implants. The improvement is very noticeable.

Breast Augmentation Scar Healing

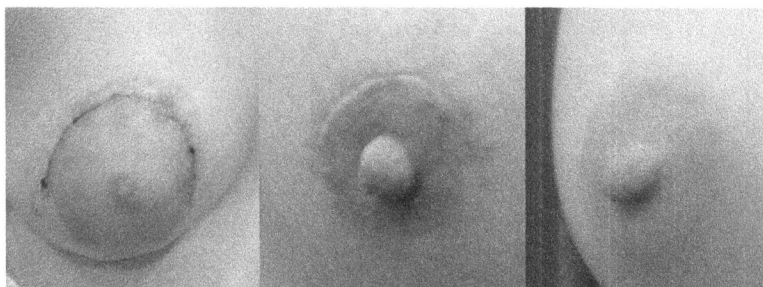

| **Very fresh periareolar incision** | **A healing periareolar incision** | **Fully healed periareolar incision** |

Breast Augmentation Gone Wrong
(other surgeons' work that Dr. Vip repaired)

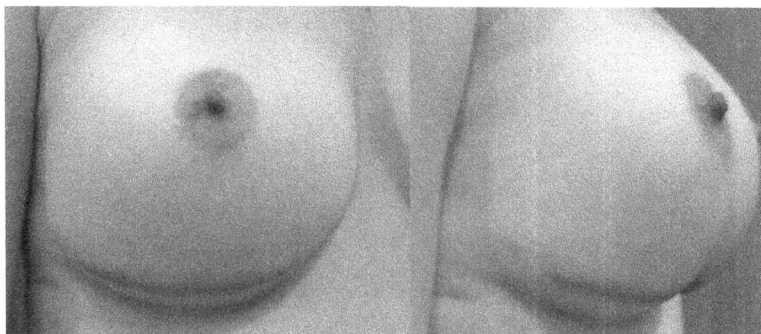

Patient 8 came to Dr. Vip with very noticeable dark scars on her breasts from a previous surgeon. This is what a bad boob job can look like. Dr. Vip fixed the scarring.

RESOURCES

Dr. Vip Dev: *www.vipmd.com* (661) 327-2101

Government Web Sites

National Institutes of Health: *www.nlm.nih.gov/medlineplus/breastimplantsbreastreconstruction.html*

FDA: *www.fda.gov.cdrh/breastimplants*

Surgical Organizations

American Board of Plastic Surgery:
www.abplsurg.org

Royal College of Physicians and Surgeons of Canada:
www.rcpsc.medical.org
American Board of Medical Specialties:
www.abms.org
American Society of Plastic Surgeons:
www.plasticsurgery.org

Implant Manufacturers

www.allergan.com

www.mentorcorp.com

Information for Her and Forums

www.BreastImplantInfo.org

www.BreastImplants4You.com

www.JustBreastImplants.com

www.BreastImplants411.com

www.ImplantForum.com

www.ImplantInfo.com

www.RealSelf.com

Other Misc.

www.BreastImplantAnswers.com (Allergan)

www.Natrelle.com (Allergan)

www.MemoryGel.com (Mentor)

www.breast-plastic-surgery.org

www.makemeheal.com